Logic of Discovery and Diagnosis in Medicine

Pittsburgh Series in
Philosophy and History
of Science

Series Editors:

Adolf Grünbaum
Larry Laudan
Nicholas Rescher
Wesley C. Salmon

Logic of Discovery
and Diagnosis
in Medicine

Edited by

Kenneth F. Schaffner

UNIVERSITY OF CALIFORNIA PRESS
Berkeley   Los Angeles   London

University of California Press
Berkeley and Los Angeles, California

University of California Press, Ltd.
London, England

Copyright © 1985 by The Regents of the University of California

Library of Congress Cataloging in Publication Data

Main entry under title:

Logic of discovery and diagnosis in medicine.

(Pittsburgh series in philosophy and history of science)
Papers originating from the Workshop on "the Logic of Discovery and Diagnosis in
Medicine" held at the University of Pittsburgh in Oct. 1978.
1. Diagnosis—Data processing—Congresses.   2. Medical logic—Congresses.
3. Medicine—Philosophy—Congresses.   4. Problem solving—Congresses.
I. Schaffner, Kenneth F.   II. Workshop on "the Logic of Discovery and Diagnosis
in Medicine" (1978 : University of Pittsburgh)   III. Series. [DNLM: 1. Com-
puters—congresses. 2. Diagnosis—congresses. 3. Diagnosis, Computer Assisted—
congresses. 4. Logic—congresses. 5. Problem Solving—congresses.
WB 141 L832]
RC71.3.L64   1985   616.07'5'02854   84–28009
ISBN 0–520–05305–2

1 2 3 4 5 6 7 8 9

Contents

Preface

The papers in this volume had their origin in a Workshop on "The Logic of Discovery and Diagnosis in Medicine" held at the University of Pittsburgh in October of 1978. The planning decisions were made by a committee composed of Kenneth F. Schaffner (Chair), William M. Cooper, Adolf Grünbaum, Larry Laudan, Jack D. Myers, and Harry E. Pople, Jr. Many of the papers have been extensively revised and elaborated on since the Workshop, and the Introduction to this volume indicates the place of the papers in the development of this exciting interdisciplinary field as well as provides a perspective on their relation to current research.

Grateful acknowledgment is made to the Sarah Scaife Foundation for support of the Workshop from which this volume developed, and to the Richard King Mellon Foundation for further support during the editing process. I also want to thank Thomas Detre, James Greeno, Alvin P. Shapiro, and Gerhard Werner for chairing Workshop sessions.

I also wish to express appreciation to Mary Ann Cooper for coordinating local arrangements and Jane Rodwell Carugati for editorial assistance.

Pittsburgh, Pennsylvania   Kenneth F. Schaffner
April 1985

Introduction

Kenneth F. Schaffner

This volume contains papers originally presented at a Conference on Logic of Discovery and Diagnosis in Medicine held at the University of Pittsburgh.[1] In this introduction I will provide a background for the papers and will attempt to elucidate some of the common themes that occupied the Conference. In addition to sketching a background for the Conference papers I will integrate into my remarks an "afterword" so as to situate the Conference papers within important recent developments that have taken place in philosophy of science, artificial intelligence, and the analysis of clinical diagnosis. I begin with a review of some of the common themes of the Conference and an account of the Conference's genesis.

Two of several common themes tying many of the essays together are the notions of "problem solving" and "heuristic search" as applied to discovery and diagnosis in the biomedical sciences. The Program Committee for the Conference was composed of two physicians, two philosophers, and an artificial-intelligence theorist, and was seeking some common—and, it was hoped, synergistic—ground between these disciplines. The initial motivation for such a Conference was based on three developments in philosophy of science, in medicine, and in artificial intelligence, respectively. First, the 1960s and 1970s witnessed the beginnings of a general revival of interest in the notion of a "logic of scientific discovery" in philosophy of science. This revival was primarily intiated by Hanson's work.[2] The ferment in philosophy of science following the attacks on logical empiricism and the development of a viable alternative approach by Kuhn, Feyerabend, and Toulmin, among others, contributed to a willingness to reexamine the subject.[3] The publication of the two volumes edited by Nickles in 1980 on scientific discovery typifies this development.[4]

Second, medical analyses of the diagnostic process during the 1950s and 1960s had indicated that this domain was considerably more complex than initially thought. Simpler branching-logic and elementary Bayesian probability models began to be seen as incapable of capturing the rich content of medical diagnosis.[5] In the 1970s researchers in this area began to turn increasingly to the field of Artificial Intelligence (AI) in attempts to represent this task domain. An organization of researchers in this area of Artificial Intelligence in Medicine (AIM) was formed and began formal meetings in 1975.

Third, the field of artificial intelligence began to appear as a promising tool for analysts of the clinical diagnostic process. AI had begun to make significant advances in capturing problem-solving behavior and in developing searching strategies in complex subject areas. One program, DENDRAL, which was in the process of evolution at Stanford in the early 1970s, appeared to be on the way toward discovering chemical structures that would constitute publishable new knowledge in the area of organic chemistry. At Pittsburgh the clinical diagnostic program initially known as INTERNIST and now as CADUCEUS had demonstrated striking successes in diagnosing difficult patient problems.

These three reasons, with some elaboration and application to the contributions at the Conference, will constitute an appropriate introduction to the papers in this volume. I will begin with an account of developments in the AI area which may assist us in providing background for a number of the papers to follow.

AI PROBLEM SOLVING AND
HEURISTIC SEARCH

One of the contributors to this volume is Professor Herbert Simon. Simon is an economist and a psychologist as well as a philosopher of science, but we are in this introduction particularly interested in his work in artificial intelligence. In this area, which overlaps to a degree with his research in psychology, Simon has developed a theory of scientific discovery. This theory is best understood as an information-processing theory of problem solving. Simon has written that his central thesis concerning scientific discovery can be succinctly stated: "Scientific discovery is a form of problem solving, and the processes whereby science is carried on can be explained in the terms that have been used to explain the processes of problem solving" (Simon 1977, 266).

Simon's work on scientific discovery extends back approximately twenty-five years and has often been carried out in collaboration with his colleague Alan Newell. In one of their early papers, Newell and Simon introduce the crucial distinction between "finding possible solutions" and "processes for determining whether a solution proposal is in fact a solution" (Newell, Shaw, and Simon [1962] 1979, 149). Thus solution-*generating* processes are distinguished from a second class of solution-*verifying* processes. This distinction is not identical with the distinction so prominent in the literature of philosophy of science during its logical-positivistic period between the "context of discovery" and the "context of justification."[6] The latter distinction denied the applicability of logical processes to the context of discovery, whereas in Newell and Simon's work both contexts require logical analysis and representation.

Newell, Shaw, and Simon ([1962] 1979) also outline the difficulties associated with a geometrically increasing "problem maze" in which, for example, each choice point divides into two (or more) possible actions on the way toward a solution point. Trial-and-error searches through such a maze quickly become time-consuming and expensive. Successful problem solving accordingly required principles termed *heuristics* after Polya (1945), which served as guides through such mazes. Newell, Shaw, and Simon ([1962] 1979, 152) wrote: "We use the term heuristic to denote any principle or device that contributes to the reduction in the average search to solution." Such heuristics permit the problem solver, whether this be a human being or a computer, to explore only a very small part of the maze or "search space."

This notion of a "heuristic search" has served as the foundation for all later AI work in scientific discovery and in most areas of the logic of clinical diagnosis. It informs both the DENDRAL program cited above, which Bruce Buchanan's contribution discusses in detail, as well as the INTERNIST-I diagnostic program, which occupied so much of the Conference.

DIFFERENCES BETWEEN DISCOVERY
AND DIAGNOSIS PROGRAMS

In spite of these common themes between discovery and diagnosis programs, there are some significant differences. First, none of the present diagnostic programs, such as INTERNIST-I, its successor CADUCEUS, and MYCIN, attempt to diagnose *novel* diseases. If, for example, a patient with a classic case of Legionnaires' disease were to have his signs, symptoms, and laboratory data entered into INTER-NIST-I prior to the inclusion of that disease entity in its knowledge base, INTERNIST-I would not be able to diagnose the disease. Neither the INTERNIST-I program nor any other diagnostic program with which I am familiar can generate a concept of a *new* disease. Such programs can, however, diagnose simultaneous or concurrent aggregates of diseases which may never have been seen previously. The situation as regards novelty generation in discovery programs is less clear and more controversial. In describing the operation of the generator in DENDRAL Buchanan writes:

> The DENDRAL generator of molecular structures (named CONGEN for Constrained Generator) is the heart of the whole program. The problem description it starts with is a list of chemical atoms (including the number of atoms of each type) together with constraints on the ways groups of atoms can and cannot be associated. The language in which hypotheses are expressed, and generated, is the so-called "ball-and-stick" language of chemical atoms and bonds. . . .
>
> CONGEN produces a complete and nonredundant list of molecular structures containing exactly the specified atoms and satisfying the specified constraints. . . .
>
> The *unconstrained* algorithm [my emphasis] has been proved to produce all possible chemical graphs with a specified composition, without duplication. Since there are hundreds of possibilities for six-atom structures, thousands for 7–8 atoms, millions and tens of millions for 15–20 atoms, the generator cannot profitably examine every possible explanation. The need for constraints is obvious. . . . (Buchanan 1985, 148–150)

What Buchanan indicates in this question is that CONGEN is importantly limited in terms of its power to generate novel hypothetical structures by the language in which the generator is written. What CONGEN does is to envisage all possibilities, in terms of permutations and combinations, of the atoms in the "ball-and-stick" language.

This limitation is more explicitly brought out by Buchanan in his discussion of the Meta-DENDRAL program. Of this he writes:

> The Meta-DENDRAL program is designed to aid chemists find and
> explain regularities in a collection of data. . . . Although the most rev-
> olutionary discoveries involve postulating new theoretical entities (i.e.,
> developing a new theory), finding general rules is also a creative activity
> within an existing theory. It is at this level of scientific activity that the
> Meta-DENDRAL program operates. It does not postulate new terms but
> tries to find new regularities and explain them with rules written in the
> predefined vocabulary. (Buchanan 1985, 150–151)

This limitation drew criticism at the Conference from Carl G. Hempel, who commented on Buchanan's paper. Hempel wrote:

> The formulation of powerful explanatory principles, and especially
> theories, normally involves the introduction of a novel conceptual and
> terminological apparatus. The explanation of combustion by the conflict-
> ing theories of dephlogistication and of oxidation illustrates the point.
>   The new concepts introduced by a theory of this kind cannot, as a
> rule, be defined by those previously available. . . . It does not seem clear
> at all how a computer might be programmed to discover such powerful
> theories. (Hempel 1985, 179–180)

Hempel's objection concerning novelty may have been met by other
discovery programs not explicitly reviewed at the Pittsburgh Conference. A mathematical discovery program developed by Lenat (1977),
termed AM, appears to generate novel concepts in the domain of
arithmetic. Hempel could, however, easily reply that discovery in
mathematics is fundamentally different from discovery in the natural
sciences, since the former is logically analytic whereas the latter involves moves that require ampliative inference. (In ampliative inference, the conclusion possesses more "content" than is implicit in the
premises.)

Of probably greater force against Hempel's objection is the discovery program developed by Langley working closely with Simon and
his colleagues. This program is known as BACON, and it has gone
through several revisions in the past few years. The form I shall briefly
comment on is termed the BACON.4 version.

Simon, Langley, and Bradshaw (1981, 12) claim that "BACON.4
employs a small set of data-driven heuristics to detect regularities in
numeric and nominal data. These heuristics, by noting constancies and
trends, cause BACON.4 to formulate hypotheses, define theoretical
terms, postulate intrinsic properties, and postulate integral relations
(common divisors) among quantities." This program has had one of
its heuristics applied to data of the type that may have been available

to Kepler and has generated Kepler's third law: period^2 $\propto$ (distance from sun)^3. Further, by using its "postulating-intrinsic-properties" heuristic, BACON.4 makes an attempt to reply to Hempel's comment that new theoretical properties cannot be generated by a computer-based discovery program. It would take us beyond the scope of this introduction to analyze the arguments of Simon, Langley, and Bradshaw on this point, and their 1981 article should be consulted by the interested reader; suffice it to say that the debate concerning discovery of novel properties, novel entities, and, *a fortiori,* novel diseases is not closed and continues to generate both research and controversy.

THE LOGIC OF MEDICAL DIAGNOSIS

Most of the papers in this volume constitute an introduction to the logic of medical diagnosis and to various computer implementations of that logic. These issues involve philosophical problems as well as difficult problems in the AI field. In addition, the discipline to which philosophy and AI are applied, medicine, poses its own problems to the clinician, such as disease classification and definition. In this and the next two sections I will summarize and review the contributions of Clouser, Kyburg, Engelhardt, Simon, Myers, and Pople to the Conference; I will also touch on the comments of McMullin, Suppe, and Seidenfeld which are relevant to these papers. I will begin in this section with an overview of some of the issues that arise in the context of clinical diagnosis. In the following two sections I will outline the INTERNIST-I program that was extensively discussed at the Conference, and then turn to some of the problems with INTERNIST-I and steps that are currently being taken to solve these problems.

Feinstein (1969) succinctly represents the relation between nature's path and the doctor's reasoning in the following diagram:[7]

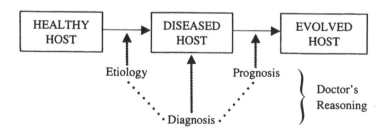

In a later essay Feinstein notes that diagnostic reasoning is the "process of converting observed evidence into the names of diseases. The *evidence* consists of data obtained from examining a patient; the *diseases* are conceptual medical entities that identify or explain abnormalities in the observed evidence" (1973, 212). This simple diagram and definition of diagnostic reasoning will serve to introduce Clouser's, Kyburg's, Engelhardt's, and Simon's contributions to the Conference.

K. Danner Clouser's task in his paper is to "approach diagnosis very broadly and very gently." This is intended to bring a diverse group of philosophers, physicians, and artificial-intelligence theorists to the point where they have a common, if introductory, comprehension of the diagnostic-reasoning process and some of the models that have been proposed to represent that process. Later papers provide more details of these models as well as criticisms of them.

Clouser begins by discussing what a physician does during the "work-up" of a patient. This involves both the gathering of information, or "data" as Feinstein refers to it, *and* an attempt to see a pattern or constellation in those data. This pattern-seeing is an attempt to place the patient in a *classification* because "the physician's knowledge of causes, treatment, and prognoses are organized that way." This physician's reasoning involves various judgments that the patient has certain diseases. Such judgments represent probabilistic thinking in which there are certain recurring elements. Clouser introduces us subtly to these elements usually termed *prior probabilities* and *likelihoods,* and before we are aware of it he has provided us with an intuitive understanding of the way in which these elements fit together into what is termed *Bayes' theorem.*

Bayes' theorem is a formal theorem of the axiomatized probability calculus, and *as such* is reasonably uncontroversial. The theorem has several forms, but perhaps the simplest (following Wulff 1981, 85) is

$$P(D|C) = \frac{P(C|D)\ P(D)}{P(C)}$$

where $P(D|C)$ is the posterior probability and refers to the probability of the patient's having the disease D given symptom C, $P(C|D)$ is the likelihood of a patient's exhibiting C given that he has D, $P(D)$ is the prior probability that the patient has D, and $P(C)$ is the probability that the patient will exhibit C whether or not he has D. When the theorem is given an interpretation and applied either in statistical reasoning or in the logic of diagnosis, it leads both to problems and to controversies. Clouser discusses some of these limitations of the "Bayesian" approach, which makes extensive use of Bayes' theorem in modeling diagnostic reasoning. Other papers at the Conference, particularly the contributions of Kyburg and Seidenfeld, also make reference to this approach and its difficulties, and an extensive further literature can be consulted by the interested reader.[8]

Clouser also considers the question of the "overall structure" of diagnostic reasoning. He notes that some have proposed that it is a kind of branching logic. The extent to which a branching logic is a feasible representation of diagnostic logic is considered by several of the contributors to the conference with different conclusions. We will return to this issue again below.

One topic introduced by Clouser involves the nature of the disease entities that are the end points of diagnosis. As noted above, such end points are construed as a "classification." Clouser raises the question of how fine a structure we need in our disease classification in order to arrive at a diagnosis that will permit appropriate prognosis and treatment. He worries about, but does not propose a solution to, the increase in complexity which consideration of the *stages* of a disease may introduce into diagnostic reasoning calculations. This is an issue that is not at all settled and that may require further developments in AI to deal with because of its computational and logical complexity.

Henry Kyburg's paper follows on from Clouser's introductory account and examines the general nature of inductive logic and some of the assumptions that are made in medical reasoning. Kyburg situates inductive logic within logic in general and reminds us, in an unfortunate contrast with deductive logic, that "there is no widespread agreement on *what inductive logic is,* or on *the sense of probability involved,* or even on *how it is supposed to function*" (1985, 187). Kyburg's paper represents a series of arguments and suggestions addressed to these three points.

Kyburg's answer begins with the second problem, that is, with an examination of the sense of *probability* that might be involved. Here he develops his own notion of an "epistemological" interpretation of probability. This interpretation is partly "logical," in the sense that there is an important linguistic component to it, but it is also "frequentist" to the extent that "every probability corresponds to a *known* relative frequency or measure. . . ." This latter idea of a relative frequency implicitly introduces the notion of a reference class (1985, 192). Correlative with the notion of a reference class is the concept of randomness, which for Kyburg is also an epistemological notion. The common idea behind these notions is that we select the reference class in which to place an individual about whom we wish to make a (clinical) prediction on the basis of all the relevant knowledge we have. Then within the reference classes, individuals thus described will behave as random elements with respect to predictions of the (clinical) property under consideration.

Kyburg applies these notions to several epidemiological examples. One particularly interesting argument he presents is that a pure frequency approach to randomness will not do for medical epidemiology. Kyburg also examines the relations between his epistemological approach to probability and the kinds of belief changes that occur when Bayes' theorem is applied. (These belief changes are often referred to as "conditionalization" because of the use of conditional probability in the expression for posterior probability.) Kyburg points out, as Clouser and others did as well, that a Bayesian approach to diagnosis generally assumes independence of the manifestations of a disease. This is implausible, and thus Bayesians feel the need to test for independence. Surprisingly, some Bayesians (e.g., Nugent et al. 1964) abandon the Bayesian framework and test for independence using a χ^2 test. Kyburg notes that though this may be intuitively appealing, it is not justified on Bayesian grounds. He sketches an argument to show that his epistemological notion of probability can incorporate such moves under certain specified conditions. Kyburg also has some additional interesting comments on the role of probability in INTERNIST-I which I shall postpone until we have reviewed that program.

In his paper Teddy Seidenfeld examines several of Kyburg's claims by first construing Kyburg's position as a kind of Fisherian compromise between the Bayesians and the orthodox classical school of hypothesis-testing followed by most biostaticians. Seidenfeld argues that different positions on conditionalization taken by the orthodox approach, by Kyberg and the Fisherians, and by the Bayesians lead to three different verdicts on randomization. For the Bayesians, Seidenfeld sketches a formal proof showing that on the assumption of Bayesian conditionalization, randomization is irrelevant. For Kyburg, randomization may make sense pretrial or posttrial, but may not be required. Seidenfeld argues that this decision is exactly dependent on whether conditionalization is licensed. For orthodox statisticians, for whom conditionalization is invalid whenever a "prior" probability is inappropriate, randomization is required.

Kyburg's paper and Seidenfeld's comments suggest that the logic of medical diagnosis will find further research in inductive logic to be of considerable value. Several additional comments by both Kyburg and Seidenfeld that refer to current work in inductive logic but touch directly on INTERNIST-I will be considered further below.

In connection with the diagram from Feinstein introduced above, I indicated that disease classifications are essential to the diagnostic reasoning process. Unfortunately, just as there is no consensus in the area of inductive logic, there is no firm consensus on a disease classification, though a number of attempts have been made. In his paper, H. Tristram Engelhardt, Jr. explores the foundations of the disease concept and the typology of disease notion. He provides us with a brief history of disease classification and also examines the philosophical question of the value-free nature of the disease concept. The tie-in between this latter question and the classification problem is significant: if the disease concept is nonnormative, it is more likely that a consensus can be reached concerning a disease classification. If on the other hand the disease concept is value-laden, there are likely to be many different, even idiosyncratic classifications reflecting different individuals' and societies' values in addition to the descriptive content in a disease classification.

Though it will probably lead to increased diversity and complexity, Engelhardt tends to favor the value-laden interpretation of the disease concept. In addition, he follows Wulff (1976) in arguing for various alternative typologies of diseases, "aimed at facilitating different sorts of clinical decision-making." For Wulff, diseases are vehicles of clinical knowledge and experience, and the main function of a disease category is to further better treatment. The moral that can be drawn from Engelhardt's paper is that the physician, logician, or AI theorist should proceed *flexibly* in approaching the issues of disease definition and disease classification, depending on the purposes of the classification. For Wulff and Engelhardt, most physicians aim at diagnostic efficiency as a prelude to maximizing therapeutic effectiveness. A proposal for classification flexibility does not, of course, license a wholesale rejection of traditional disease definitions and typologies. That would almost certainly lead to a useless, and ignored, classification with the same probable fate awaiting the AI theorist's program that employed such a radical nonstandard classification. On this view, however, researchers pursuing the modeling of diagnostic logics are free to reconfigure diagnostic classification in the interest of logical efficiency if they factor in the trade-offs with the easier acceptability that a familiar definition and/or classification would yield. In the section below headed "Parallel Processing, Tangled Hierarchical Classification, and CADUCEUS," we shall see just how important the pursuit of a somewhat novel and flexible classification system has become to more recent developments in CADUCEUS.

Achieving a diagnosis requires not only an adequate set of disease definitions and a disease classification but also, as Feinstein notes in his diagram above, a reasoning process that will take the doctor from patient data *to* a disease. In discussing Clouser's essay I have already introduced some features of this reasoning process, and Herbert Simon in his paper takes the discussion further.

Simon brings his considerable knowledge of AI and its techniques to bear on the issues of clinical diagnosis and the possible modeling of the diagnostic process by a computer. Just as scientific discovery was construed under a "problem solving" rubric, Simon approaches diagnoses as instances of problem solving. Following Newell and Simon 1972, he writes:

> The usual definition of a problem runs like this: Given a set U, to find a member of a subset of U having specified properties (called the goal set, G). As a first approximation in the case of medical diagnosis, we can take U as the set of all possible disease entities, G as the disease present in a particular patient (or the collection of his diseases, if he has more than one), and the "specified properties" as the indications, for example, a pathologist would use on autopsy to determine what the disease "really was." (Simon 1985, 114–115)

Diagnosis under this approach involves, as do the Feinstein and Clouser analyses, a mapping of symptoms (and other patient data) onto a disease(s).

Given a disease classification or taxonomy, Simon suggests that we can construe diagnosis as an analogue of the "twenty questions" game: "construct a taxonomic key that prompts the user down a branching list of questions the answers to which discriminate successively among groups of species until a unique identification has been made" (1985, 116). This is, Simon notes, a first approximation that will need to be modified in the light of other features of the diagnostic process. The unreliability and noisiness of the data require that we understand the linkages in the branching tree to be probabilistic. This in turn suggests that we interpret the branching process as a problem in statistical decision theory which generally will make extensive use of Bayes' theorem, which was introduced above. The Bayesian account has, as was noted earlier, several severe limitations. Simon is aware of these and concludes that a Bayesian approach is better conceived of as a "guide" to the general shape of a diagnostic program. There are other useful features of a Bayesian decision-theoretic analysis which Simon comments on, such as an ability to factor in the costs of errors.

A branching-logic analysis of the diagnostic process, even one supplemented with probabilistic considerations, is not, however, entirely satisfactory to Simon. It leaves out a key element, namely a "reasoned account of the relation between symptoms and disease." One way to import a more intelligent approach to diagnosis into our model is to conceive symptoms as being *caused* by diseases. These causal links would presumably replace the correlation links found in the more nosological approach discussed initially. (As we shall see further below, it is possible to consider the nosological and the causal approaches to the relation between diseases and symptoms as *overlapping* rather than as exclusive.) Under the causal approach one proceeds not by an elimination of branches nor by a Bayesian comparison of branches but rather by a "hypothesize-and-test" methodology. This is a feature of the CADUCEUS approach and will be discussed in the following section.

The causal construal of disease-symptom linkages suggests to Simon an analogy with a (primitive) model of the etiology of disease. Such a model would be both rather crude and quite abstract, but it might reflect fairly accurately a kind of "commonsense" reasoning system. In contrast with this crude system, Simon proposes that we consider, as a rather different approach to diagnosis, a rather sophisticated and quantitative model that has been used to diagnose malfunctions in electronic circuits. This is the SOPHIE program developed by Bobrow and Brown (1975). Simon suggests that though there are difficulties with causal modeling and with the logics used to represent causal linkages, this seems a most promising approach to diagnostic reasoning. He provides several other examples in his paper of "trouble-shooting" and "causal-localization" programs. It should be added that other AI investigators have emphasized the causal features of medical diagnosis. See for example Weiss and Kulikowski's CASNET program

(Weiss et al. 1978) and Patil, Szolovitz, and Schwartz's (1981) ABEL program.

Simon closes his paper urging that a systematic evaluation of diagnostic programs be undertaken. This would involve an examination of the effect of increasing the knowledge base of diagnostic programs, as well as an in-depth comparative assessment of different basic methods such as the twenty-questions, statistical-decision-theory, and causal-linkage schemes. He also makes a most interesting suggestion, which in a way is being taken up in current research on CADUCEUS, that we need to model more human anatomy and physiology in diagnostic programs. Such modeling need *not* be fully detailed fine-structure anatomy and physiology; it could well be that "we would extract from the models their important qualitative properties and convert these into systems of causal linkages that we could incorporate into our diagnostic-reasoning schemes" (1985, 135). A number of Simon's proposals are most insightful, and we will return to and reexamine them below in the light of current diagnostic-reasoning developments.

At this point I have introduced the concept of diagnostic reasoning and related it to several general approaches in AI. I now turn to an overview of a computer-based diagnostic program which illustrates many of the approaches as well as problems that have been touched on above. This is the INTERNIST-I diagnostic program that occupied much of the Conference's discussion.

AN OVERVIEW OF INTERNIST-I

INTERNIST-I is a clinical diagnostic program in internal medicine which utilizes the techniques of Artificial Intelligence (AI). It was developed by Jack Myers, a distinguished internist, and Harry Pople, a computer scientist, beginning in 1974. In a very real sense the INTERNIST-I program is an AI partial simulation of Jack Myers's clinical-reasoning processes and his own internal knowledge-base. (Myers is known to mildly grimace, however, when INTERNIST-I is referred to as "Jack-in-the-box.") Randy Miller, a physician, soon joined the project, along with several programmers and (over the years) a number of medical students. The initial approach of Myers and Pople was, as Myers notes in his essay in this volume, toward extensive pathophysiological modeling and explanation. This turned out, relatively quickly, to be "extremely costly and often wasteful" as a procedure, and in 1975 attention was redirected toward the type of program to be described in more detail below and in the papers in this volume. It should be noted, however, that current research on the successor to INTERNIST-I termed CADUCEUS involves to an extent a return to a pathophysiological emphasis. I shall have more to say about this in a subsequent section.

The summary description of the INTERNIST-I program I shall provide in this Introduction follows essentially the contributions of Myers and Pople to this volume. I shall occasionally supplement those papers with material that was either distributed to Conference participants in advance or presented in discussion and goes into somewhat more detail on the technical and logical aspects of the INTERNIST-I program. These details have been published elsewhere but are included here for convenience.[9]

An overview of the INTERNIST-I program should begin by mentioning its extensive knowledge base. This comprises about five hundred diseases known to internal medicine that are arranged in a disease hierarchy, that is, from the general to the specific. The individual disease is the basic element in the knowledge base. Each disease is characterized by a disease profile, which is a list of manifestations—that is, signs, symptoms, and laboratory abnormalities—associated with that disease. Each manifestation in a disease profile has two clinical variables associated with it: an "evoking strength" and a "frequency." The evoking strength is a rough measure on a scale of 0 to 5 of how strongly this manifestation suggests this disease as its cause. Table 1 (from Miller, Pople, and Myers 1982) contains an interpretation of these numbers, and Tables 1 and 2 in Myers's essay in this volume provide examples of a fragment of a disease profile as well as a set of contrasting diseases evoked by a manifestation. The frequency, on the other hand, is a rough measure of how often patients with the disease have that manifestation. This is measured on a 1-through-5 scale, an interpretation of which is given in Table 2. The crudeness of the scale is demanded because of the unreliability of data in internal medicine. The medical literature is the source for frequency numbers, though again because of the quality of the data a judgmental element figures in as well. In addition to these two numbers each manifestation is assigned an "import" on a scale of 1 through 5 as interpreted in Table 3. The import is a disease-*independent* measure of the global importance of explaining that manifestation.

TABLE 1. INTERPRETATION OF EVOKING STRENGTHS

Evoking Strength	Interpretation
0	Nonspecific—manifestation occurs too commonly to be used to construct a differential diagnosis
1	Diagnosis is a rare or unusual cause of listed manifestation
2	Diagnosis causes a substantial minority of instances of listed manifestation
3	Diagnosis is the most common but not the overwhelming cause of listed manifestation
4	Diagnosis is the overwhelming cause of listed manifestation
5	Listed manifestation is pathognomonic for the diagnosis

TABLE 2. INTERPRETATION OF FREQUENCY VALUES

Frequency	Interpretation
1	Listed manifestation occurs rarely in the disease
2	Listed manifestation occurs in a substantial minority of cases of the disease
3	Listed manifestation occurs in roughly half the cases
4	Listed manifestation occurs in the substantial majority of cases
5	Listed manifestation occurs in essentially all cases—i.e., it is a prerequisite for the diagnosis

In addition to the disease profiles with their manifestations, INTERNIST-I also contains "links" between diseases, about 2,600 at present, which are meant to capture the degree to which one disease may cause or predispose to another. There are also approximately another 6,500 relations among manifestations as well; for example, "sex: female" is a precondition of "oligomenorrhea."

INTERNIST-I contains a number of problem-solving algorithms that operate on the individual-patient data entered, using the information contained in the knowledge base. In order to follow the application of these somewhat abstract algorithms, the reader is encouraged to consult Myers's specific case example of progressive systemic sclerosis

TABLE 3. INTERPRETATION OF IMPORT VALUES

Import	Interpretation
1	Manifestation is usually unimportant, occurs commonly in normal persons, and is easily disregarded
2	Manifestation may be of importance, but can often be ignored; context is important
3	Manifestation is of medium importance, but may be an unreliable indicator of any specific disease
4	Manifestation is of high importance and can only rarely be disregarded as, for example, a false-positive result
5	Manifestation absolutely must be explained by one of the final diagnoses

Source: Tables from Miller, Pople, and Myers 1982 defining evoking strength, frequency, and import.

involving the kidney presented in his paper. In this Introduction I shall concentrate on the general problem-solving procedures and the logic of the program's reasoning process.

As a specific case with the patient's manifestations is entered into the computer, the INTERNIST-I program generates disease hypotheses that may account for that manifestation. This is a simple and direct triggering process that employs the lists contained in the knowledge base linking manifestations to diseases. Myers's Table 2 is an illustration of how this works. This set of disease hypotheses, which is usually huge, is termed the master list. In addition, for *each* disease hypothesis four associated lists are maintained that represent the match and lack of match between the specific patient under consideration and the disease profile. Myers's essay describes these lists in detail.

Each disease hypothesis on the master list is assigned a score on the basis of the match between the patient's set of manifestations and the knowledge-base disease profiles. Counting in favor of a specific disease hypothesis are the manifestations explained by that hypothesis. Credit is awarded on the basis of the manifestations' evoking strengths. Counting against a specific disease are (1) manifestations expected but found absent in the specific patient, which are debited in terms of the frequency values, and (2) manifestations not accounted for by the disease hypothesis, which are debited in accord with the import of that manifestation. In addition, a bonus is awarded to any disease that is related to a previously diagnosed disease via links in the knowledge base. This bonus is equal to twenty times the frequency number associated with the hypothesized disease in the previously diagnosed disease's profile.

A disease's total score is based on a nonlinear weighting scheme that differs for scores based on evoking strengths, frequencies, and imports. Such nonlinearity has often been found in descriptive studies of human judgment in a variety of disciplines, and thus should not be a surprising feature of INTERNIST-I.[10] The weighting scheme assigns "points" in the following fashion:[11]

(i) for evoking strengths: $0 = 1, 1 = 4, 2 = 10, 3 = 20,$
    $4 = 40, 5 = 80$

(ii) for frequencies: $1 = -1, 2 = -4, 3 = -7, 4 = -15, 5 = -30$

(iii) for imports: $1 = -2, 2 = -6, 3 = -10, 4 = -20, 5 = -40,$

in accord with the crediting/debiting procedure mentioned in the previous paragraph. These nonlinear point assignments represent Myers's clinical judgment as honed by continuing experience with the INTERNIST-I program applied to patient cases.

All the disease hypotheses on the master list are scored in accordance with the procedure outlined in the two previous paragraphs. Then the topmost set of hypotheses above a threshold is processed further by a simple but powerful sorting heuristic that partitions this topmost set into natural competing sets of disease hypotheses. This allows INTERNIST-I, as Myers notes, to compare "apples with apples and oranges with oranges." This sorting heuristic can be stated in various ways. One recent formulation is: "Two diseases are competitors if the items not explained by one disease are a subset of the items not explained by the other; otherwise they are alternatives (and may possibly coexist in the patient)" (Miller, Pople, and Myers 1982, 471). This idea can be put another way by realizing that two different diseases, A and B, that meet this criterion will, if taken together, not explain any more of the manifestations than either one does taken alone. This sorting heuristic thus creates a "current problem area" consisting of the highest ranked disease hypothesis and its competitors. Miller, Pople, and Myers (1982, 471) refer to this procedure for defining a problem area as "*ad hoc,*" and note that because of the procedure, INTERNIST-I's "differential diagnoses will not always resemble those constructed by clinicians." This, it will turn out, is a *critical* difficulty for the program and is a point to which I shall return below.

At this point INTERNIST-I will either conclude with a diagnosis or commence with one of its interactive searching modes. A diagnosis is concluded if the leading disease hypothesis is 90 points higher than its nearest competitor. This value was selected because it is just a bit more than the "absolute" weight assigned to a pathognomonic manifestation.[12] It should be stressed here that this method of concluding a diagnosis is *comparative* with respect to its competitors as defined by the sorting heuristic and is not based on any absolute probabilistic threshold, such as >0.9. If a diagnosis is not concludable, INTERNIST-I enters one of its searching modes.

In a searching mode, additional information is requested from the user. The specific mode that is entered, and thus the type of question posed, is determined by the number of competitors within 45 points of the leading diagnosis. If there is none, then INTERNIST-I enters the *Pursue* mode, posing specific questions to the user which have a high evoking strength for the topmost hypothesis. If the answer is yes to these questions, the program will rapidly reach a conclusion. If, however, there are a number of competing hypotheses running neck and neck, specifically five or more within 45 points of the leading diagnosis, the program enters its *Rule-out* mode. Here questions that have high frequency values for the competitors are asked of the user, the rationale being that negative answers will result in the rapid elimination of some of the contending hypotheses. Finally, if two to four hypotheses cluster within 45 points of the leading diagnosis, the program enters its *Discriminate* mode. Here questions are posed to the user which are likely to yield answers that would increase the separation in scores between or among the competing hypotheses.

An examination of the patient case in Myers's paper will disclose that several questions are asked at a time and that the program then recalculates its scores; it may well also repartition its diagnostic hypotheses. Questioning proceeds from the more easily obtained data to the more expensive and invasive information. Once a diagnosis is concluded, the manifestations accounted for by that diagnosis are *removed from further consideration*. This is an important point that should be noted; I will comment on it again in connection with some of its deleterious consequences. If there are manifestations that are not accounted for, the program recycles and by this process can diagnose multiple coexisting diseases.

There are two circumstances in which INTERNIST-I will terminate without reaching a diagnosis. First, if all questions have been exhausted and a conclusion has not been reached, the program will "defer" and terminate with a differential diagnosis in which the competitors are displayed and ranked in descending order. Second, if all the unexplained manifestations have an import of 2 or less, the program stops.

INTERNIST-I is a powerful program, surprisingly so in the light of its prima facie "brute-force" methods of analyzing clinical data. A formal evaluation of its diagnostic prowess by Miller, Pople, and Myers (1982) indicates that its performance is "qualitatively similar to that of the hospital clinicians but inferior to that of the [expert] case discussants." The program does, however, possess a number of problems on which work continues to be done. These problems are pointed out in the papers by Myers and Pople and also in the comments of McMullin and Suppe. Here I will only rehearse the main difficulties with INTERNIST-I in order to indicate the direction of research done since the Conference and what problems are the focus of investigations still in the future.

CRITIQUES OF INTERNIST-I; INTERNIST-II AS AN "UNSTABLE INTERMEDIATE"

In spite of the striking performance of INTERNIST-I noted in the previous section, its developers have felt since even before the Conference that fundamental further refinements were needed in the program. It should be stressed, however, that in artificial intelligence in medicine, it is relatively easy to articulate criticisms and very difficult to implement systemic corrections. In part this is so because of the impact any change has on other aspects of the program.

Pople's paper, after indicating the limitations of both the Bayesian and branching-logic approaches and giving an overview of INTERNIST-I, provides a critique of the program. One difficulty is pragmatic but nonetheless very important, namely the inappropriate initial focus of INTERNIST-I in complex problems. As Pople notes, this rarely leads to false conclusions, but the amount of time the user is required to spend at the terminal and the number of questions asked would lead to user nonacceptance. This seems to be a consequence of the scoring procedure, which provides higher scores for unifying disease hypotheses even if two distinct hypotheses might both account for the data better and lead to a diagnostic conclusion faster. This intuition set the stage for a temporary successor system known as INTERNIST-II, on which I shall comment below.

The papers by McMullin and Suppe, both philosophers of science, also contain criticisms, or at least caveats, for INTERNIST's developers. The contributions of Kyburg and Seidenfeld, it has also been mentioned, have some observations if not criticisms to make about INTERNIST-I. I shall mention some of McMullin's, Kyburg's, and Seidenfeld's points here, since they are primarily directed at INTERNIST-I (though those comments which are more relevant for other issues will be temporarily deferred); I shall review Suppe's comments that are more concerned with INTERNIST-II and CADUCEUS toward the end of this section.

McMullin's comments are far-ranging, and in this already rather long Introduction I shall be able to touch on only a few. First, I want to draw the reader's attention to McMullin's concern with the scoring algorithm in INTERNIST-I. Recall that manifestations present in the patient but not accounted for by the disease being scored count *against* that disease, the specific penalty being a function of the "import" weights of those unexplained manifestations. McMullin is troubled by this and notes that it "seems very odd." He writes: "After all, a second co-occurrent disease may very well explain the residue of the manifestations left untouched by the original D[isease]-hypothesis. So the fact that D does not account for that group of manifestations ought not, logically speaking, to count against the first D-hypothesis" (1985, 294). McMullin seems to be urging that the residue class ought to be neutral in some respect as regards the first disease hypothesis. This appears to be yet another way, in addition to Pople's observation noted above, in which INTERNIST-I's scoring algorithm is heavily biased toward a unifying disease hypothesis.

McMullin introduces several other concerns about INTERNIST-I. He notes that the clustering or partitioning procedure is "not quite clear" (1985, 300). I think this is not the case in one sense, since the sorting heuristic discussed in the previous section seems quite straightforward. But there is a more fundamental issue with which McMullin seems concerned, namely the homology or structural similarity of the manifestation lists between diseases. How this might influence the diagnostic process is a complex issue to which I shall return below. McMullin is also worried by the serial-processing aspect of INTERNIST-I, recommending a parallel-processing approach. This seems similar to Pople's INTERNIST-II methodology and will be reviewed later.

McMullin mentions two other "shortcomings" of INTERNIST-I. First, INTERNIST-I does not have the capacity to represent the *temporal* development of a patient's illness. This is, I believe, generally acknowledged to be a fundamental problem with INTERNIST-I, and its solution is not yet clear. Second, McMullin accepts Whitbeck's (1981) criticism that INTERNIST-I is too weighted toward diagnosis in contrast with therapy. To McMullin, INTERNIST-I "could do more," the "more" being a first-order-of-business review of the patient's problem to investigate any especially life-threatening illness, and also to disregard (temporarily) any alternative disease for which no therapy is available. It seems to me that though the first recommendation is laudable, the second is methodologically unsound, since it assumes an answer before the investigation has sufficiently run its course.[13] It should be added, however, that McMullin's main concern here is that it might be helpful to have a means available to the clinician using INTERNIST to permit him or her to temporarily override the normal heuristic to pursue possible high-rated leads (personal communication).

Criticisms of INTERNIST-I in addition to those mentioned have appeared in the literature, some of the most forceful by the developers themselves. Miller, Pople, and Myers (1982) note that INTERNIST-I cannot reason causally (its link structure excepted) and accordingly cannot provide appropriate explanations. In addition, it does not handle the interdependency of manifestations well, which probably will require a more causally structured knowledge base for a solution. The program is also deficient in that it has no anatomical knowledge and "cannot recognize subcomponents of an illness such as specific organ-system involvements or the degree of severity of pathologic processes" (1982, 474).

In what are not so much criticisms as suggestions for further consideration, both Kyburg and Seidenfeld focused on the numerical features of the INTERNIST-I knowledge base. Kyburg points out that, in contrast with the language of INTERNIST-I's developers, the notion of frequencies actually plays a larger role. He suggests that empirical knowledge may eventually affect evoking strengths and observes that imports and frequencies do not function entirely independently in INTERNIST-I because of the scoring algorithm. Seidenfeld notes that a curious result in inductive logic known as "Stein's paradox" suggests that more precise inductive knowledge of the frequencies in INTERNIST-I may be obtained by a global consideration of all the frequency relations at once. Seidenfeld does not provide a specific means of implementing this suggestion, though it does seem a provocative one.

A recurrent criticism, mentioned earlier in this section, relates to the *serial processing of a problem area generated by the existing scoring algorithm and partitioning heuristic*. A careful examination of the terms contained in the italicized part of the previous sentence will indicate how close to the heart of INTERNIST-I this criticism lies. At least two attempts have been made to deal with this problem, which has several different facets. At the Conference, Pople discussed a successor to INTERNIST-I that was termed INTERNIST-II. This program was implemented, and it dealt with some complex cases rather well. Pople describes INTERNIST-II in his paper, to which I now briefly turn.

INTERNIST-II's primary goal was to develop a methodology for *concurrent* problem-formulation. To this end, Pople introduced several new concepts into the INTERNIST program. First, a notion of a *constrictor* was developed as a generalization of the idea of a pathognomonic manifestation. A constrictor was invoked as a tool for generating multiple hypotheses. Pople wrote: "If the focus of attention is directed at higher levels of the disease hierarchy rather than at the terminal-level nodes, quite specific associations between very commonplace manifestations and these higher-level disease descriptors can often be established. For example, . . . bloody sputum, while not pathognomonic with respect to any particular lung problem, provides ample justification for serious consideration of the lung area as a problem focus" (1985, 271). Second, Pople used this notion of a constrictor to develop a multiproblem generator involving a modified scoring algorithm. The technical details will not be presented in this Introduction but can be found in Pople's paper in this volume. Third, Pople introduced a procedure for handling a combination of two (or more) interdependent disease hypotheses as a unitary hypothesis. Terming a single-disease solution to a patient's illness a simplex, Pople defined a *synthesis* operator that "maps partially expanded hypothesis states into new states wherein two or more *simplex* nodes have been combined into a single *complex* node. The basis for such combinations is the existence of causal, temporal, or other known patterns of associations among members of these simplex-problem sets" (1985, 275).

The reader can compare a specific patient problem analyzed without this synthesis operator with a run of INTERNIST-II employing the operator in Pople's paper. The new strategy using these new notions of constrictor, multiproblem generator, and synthesis operator appeared quite promising, and work on this approach to a successor to INTERNIST-I proceeded for about another year after the Conference.

Unfortunately, this tack ultimately did not prove fruitful. In his commentary Suppe cites personal communication from Pople indicating that the heuristics described in Pople's paper in this volume were not sufficiently powerful and that "in particular they 'washed out' various intermediate links such as the notion of infection which in actual medical practice play an important role in the clinical diagnostic procedure" (Suppe 1985, 316). The attempt, nonetheless, was a significant one, and constitutes an important, if unstable, intermediate (to use the chemists' language) between INTERNIST-I and the more elaborate successor known as CADUCEUS. In addition, the problems with INTERNIST-I that led to INTERNIST-II, as well as with the short-lived INTERNIST-II itself, generated some conceptually significant comments by both McMullin and Suppe that continue to have relevance to CADUCEUS. It is to these comments that I now turn.

PARALLEL PROCESSING, TANGLED HIERARCHICAL CLASSIFICATION, AND CADUCEUS

INTERNIST-II represented an attempt to develop a concurrent-problem-formulation approach clinical diagnosis. Both McMullin and Suppe appear to have been convinced by Pople's preliminary proposal in INTERNIST-II in this direction and urge that further attention be given to more in-depth "parallel processing." Suppe is the more specific in this regard. He cites the development of Fahlman's NETL system at Carnegie-Mellon University and Rieger's Z-Mob system at the University of Maryland as implementations of parallel-processing systems (Suppe 1985, nn. 9 and 10). Suppe suggests that NETL-like parallel capabilities could be utilized to pursue INTERNIST-I or INTERNIST-II search procedures more rapidly. He also maintains that more recent developments in the CADUCEUS version of a successor to INTERNIST-I reinforce his belief that parallel-processing approaches are both well suited to such an approach and also possess a "theoretical advantage" (1985, 334). This proposal, though suggestive, may be more feasible in the future than at present, when parallel-processing systems and "fifth-generation" machines become available. It is relevant to note that Pople's (1982) most recent in-depth account of CADUCEUS does not pursue this direction.

Earlier in this Introduction, in connection with a discussion of Engelhardt's paper, I noted that classification was a matter of considerable importance in the diagnostic process. Classification problems are discussed from two perspectives in the comments of McMullin and of Suppe, and the search for better approaches to classification has become a major recent thrust of research on CADUCEUS.

There are two interrelated ways that classification issues affect diagnosis in INTERNIST-I. The first has to do with the knowledge base or disease hierarchy, the second with the sorting heuristic that utilizes that knowledge base and partitions the differential diagnosis on the basis of the patient's manifestation list, the heuristic, and the topmost-scored disease hypothesis. McMullin's comments relate to this second or more individualized classification problem, and in particular to the partitioning heuristic that operates in INTERNIST-I. He believes this may bias the results of the inquiry, since the manifestation list associated with the topmost-scored disease hypothesis is used to separate the *total* manifestation list into those manifestations which have to be accounted for on the first cycle of the system and those which are assigned to a residue class to be pursued during the second or later cycles. Better, though McMullin believes it utopian at present, would be to take an approach similar to the direction Pople proposes in his essay. McMullin suggests "simultaneous consideration of all the possible partitionings of the M[anifestation]'s that would give rise to different sets of alternatives, and then a decision as to which set had the highest likelihood measure" (1985, 299).

This is, McMullin admits, barely reachable at the present time because of the immense number of alternatives that would have to be processed, and it is, moreover, unclear how to design either a weighting scheme for unexplained manifestations or a questioning format for such an approach. McMullin suggests two other possibilities regarding partitioning: one that might determine the "closeness" of two diseases on the basis of their shared manifestation lists and then use these sets of closely related diseases as the differential diagnosis for the range of data being considered, and the other involving use of the patient's manifestation list to construct sets of related manifestations that are above some similarity threshold in relation to the patient's manifestation list. These are speculative, and the difficulty is both in implementing them with an appropriate scoring system so as to measure appropriate similarities and in effectively differentiating them from the current INTERNIST-I heuristic, to which they could conceivably end up being equivalent.

Suppe's comments on classification problems tend to concentrate on the first set of issues mentioned above, namely on the knowledge base rather than on problems affecting partitioning. Suppe's views are best outlined in two stages. First, at the Conference he urged that, rather than accept a traditional set of diagnostic categories, INTERNIST-I's developers "possibly should consider generating its own suitably constrained taxonomic systems—subject to the realistic malpractice-inspired constraint that such taxonomics be relatable to standard-literature nosological categories and the appropriate treatment standards—and incorporating them into its heuristics and knowledge-base organization" (1985, 319–320).

Suppe considers using a numerical taxonomic scheme to generate a useful disease typology but rejects it after reviewing some of this approach's problems. A "fuzzy-set" strategy is also dismissed. Better, Suppe thinks, would be a kind of "adaptive reorganization" of INTERNIST-I's own knowledge base, perhaps at high levels, by employing Pople's constrictor concept. Suppe cites Holland's 1975 work in this regard, and in his later revisions was able to refer to Holland's 1980 essay on adaptive algorithms.

In point of fact, subsequent work on a successor to INTERNIST-I has tended to focus on the development of a modified taxonomical scheme. It would take us beyond the scope of this Introduction to present the details of this effort, but a few comments on quite recent and current research will be useful.

Many of the recent developmental extensions and modifications of INTERNIST-I are presented in Pople 1982. This paper indicated that INTERNIST-II has been largely superseded by the CADUCEUS system, though important advances that arose in INTERNIST-II, such as the constrictor concept, have been taken over into CADUCEUS. Of particular interest to us in this Introduction are further developments on the taxonomical front.

In his 1982 essay on CADUCEUS, Pople begins by stressing that the task of AI in medicine may well have been misconceived by many of its practitioners. Using a term developed by Simon (1973), Pople suggests that medical diagnosis is better conceptualized as an "ill-structured problem." Many AI programs seem to assume that diagnosis occurs within the context of a well-structured problem, that is, *after* we have restricted our attention to a differential diagnosis. A, if not *the,* major difficulty for Pople is to convert an ill-structured problem into a well-structured problem. Problem formulation, and problem synthesis in particular, is the key task. Pople argues that this process will require the most sophisticated representational and heuristic techniques available in the AI armamentarium.

I believe we can see the rationale for this new stress in CADUCEUS if we recall the problems with classification on which we have been focusing in this section. INTERNIST-II was developed to deal with the difficulty of an overly focused, serially processed problem area. (Recall the *ad hoc* construction of the differential diagnosis that was so central to INTERNIST-I's success as well as to its difficulties.) Concurrent problem-formation in INTERNIST-II was promising, but attempts at implementing this notion ultimately led Pople to realize that a modification of the INTERNIST-I knowledge base would be required. Some brief comments on this reorganization and the need for it will be useful.

Pople (1982) remarks that though it was initially hoped that "the necessary constrictor patterns could be extracted from the original INTERNIST-I knowledge structure using heuristic mapping rules," this, unfortunately, did not turn out to be the case. Pople notes that there are two reasons for this: "use of a strict hierarchy in INTERNIST-I for defining categories of disease which has served to make diffuse what would otherwise be strong constrictor relations; and elimination of pathophysiological detail which cannot be restored without a considerable investment of medical expertise. Both of these call for major revision to the structure of medical knowledge underlying the INTERNIST program" (1982, 151).

Pople's approach is to develop a "synergistic blend" of a causal or pathophysiological model with a nosological structure. We have commented earlier on the possibility of different nosological classifications depending on the goal(s) of the classifier. Pople (1982) proposes that a strict hierarchical classification is "too restrictive" and suggests that an alternative taxonomy using the notion of "organ system involvement" may be more appropriate. This will be a more complex typology "in which any given disease can be classified in as many descriptive categories of the nosology as are appropriate." Pople adds that "this type of acyclic graph structure, which allows any given node to have an arbitrary number of parent nodes, is sometimes referred to as a 'tangled hierarchy'" (1982, 157).

Implementing this reclassification requires several new notions that can be mentioned only briefly. A more extensive causal net must, of course, be introduced tying diseases and manifestations together. The added detail, however, may obscure a less detailed but unifying common cause. This would be unproblematic if the entire net were simultaneously processible, but traversing and probing such a net in a variety of directions is time-consuming and costly: accordingly, some new heuristics must be introduced that will facilitate searching such a network. Pople proposes a new type of link, referred to as a "generalized link" or "planning link," that he believes will make possible the "formulation of parsimonious refined differential diagnoses—in many cases permitting a single category to be selected as the scope of a manifestation (in which case the relationship is that of constrictor)" (1982, 159).

Just as Pople (1982) generalizes the constrictor concept to the more complex notion of a planning link, so he develops a generalization of the *synthesis* operator introduced in his discussion of INTERNIST-II. In CADUCEUS some six different simple synthesis operators are proposed that can be utilized in combination to synthesize various subtasks. The combination of these various simple operators together with planning links and their subpath instantiations constitutes a "generalized multistep unification operator."[14] These operators permit the synergistic blending of causal net focusing with nosological focusing. Considerable detail on these operators and their application is to be found in Pople 1982, to which the reader must be referred. It should be pointed out here, however, that there is as yet in CADUCEUS no simple and straightforward algorithmic procedure for achieving a final synthesis. A number of hints exist in accord with what was described above. Further work within the classical AI paradigm of "state search space" is needed (see Nilsson 1980 for examples). This work will need to be supplemented by a yet to be developed "high-level control program" that would implement Simon's approach to solutions of ill-structured problems.

Pople summarizes his expanded and reorganized vision of medical diagnosis and the place of CADUCEUS within a reconceptualized task domain as follows:

This new knowledge representation [in CADUCEUS] provides multiple nosologic structures, by which disease entities may be classified in as many descriptive ways as appropriate. In addition, there is provision for a representation of detailed pathophysiology, by means of a causal graph having no restriction as to level of resolution. These basic structures are supplemented by generalized links—a subset of the transitive closure of the causal graph—which provides for as rapid convergence on tentative unifying hypotheses as in INTERNIST-I, while at the same time enabling access—via a sub-path initiation mechanism—to as much detail as is available in the underlying causal graph.

This underlying result has been facilitated by means of a path unification algorithm used to combine elementary task definitions into unified complexes. As application of this synthesis operator cannot be considered irrevocable, it is necessary to envelop these heuristic maneuvers within a sophisticated control regime. Thus we have discovered within the task environment of medical diagnosis a core problem, the solution of which requires some of the most powerful methods available in the armamentarium of artificial intelligence. (Pople 1982, 183–184)

PARALLELS BETWEEN DISCOVERY AND CLINICAL DIAGNOSIS

I began this Introduction with an examination of Buchanan's and Hempel's papers and attempted to place both the logic of scientific discovery and the logic of medical diagnosis within a more general framework. That framework, which motivated the early planning of the Conference, arose out of a series of developments in philosophy of science, in artificial intelligence, and in attempts to represent clinical diagnosis which appeared to be exhibiting some common themes. For example, philosophy of science, owing largely to Hanson's influence, began to look more closely at the stages of both the generation and the *early* evaluation of scientific hypotheses, and not just at their justification subsequent to their having been fully elaborated. In a variety of AI programs these stages also had to be carefully examined, and the problem of generation and of early or preliminary evaluation addressed substantively by the programmers. In our discussion of INTERNIST-I above, we examined the stages through which that program proceeds in moving toward a diagnostic conclusion: often beginning in a *Rule-out* mode, moving through a comparative *Discriminate* mode, and then entering its *Pursue* mode. These procedures suggested to some of us that there were some deep analogies between scientific discovery processes and clinical diagnosis.[15] It appears to me that this is still the case, and, moreover, that developments in the three fields subsequent to the Conference have confirmed this early supposition.

We noted, in connection with a report on Langley and Simon's recent work, that scientific discovery programs that could postulate novel diseases are by no means ruled out of the province of AI. We also saw in association with Pople's recent developments of the CADUCEUS successor to INTERNIST-I and INTERNIST-II that Simon's suggestion that ill-structured problems may require new and powerful problem-solving techniques was taken up and employed in the context of clinical-diagnosis investigations. It is likely that further parallels between scientific discovery and clinical diagnosis will be disclosed by following this path.

I should at this point refer to an argument developed by McMullin in his paper which adds further support to this thesis and draws an important distinction within the realm of problem-solving behavior. McMullin distinguishes the kind of problem solving appropriate to the motorcycle mechanic from the activity of the research scientist. The motorcycle engine is an artifact, and its actions are fully understood. Further fundamental research on its causal interactions is not required. It can be broken down into its constituent parts and tested. Human beings, however, are not motorcycle engines, and the clinician's problem-solving activities are accordingly more complex. McMullin suggests the clinician's thought processes are much closer to those of the "research scientist" "because of the likely presence in the patient of causalities that are not fully understood" (1985, 309).

These issues that have been the subjects of the Conference and of this Introduction are by no means resolved. I hope to have given at least some of the flavor of the exciting and dynamic interactions that took place at this set of meetings by comparing and contrasting the variety of positions taken at the Conference. I also hope to have been able to relate the themes of the Conference and of the papers contained in this volume to events that have occurred since that time and to show that these articles represent an important, and synergistic, contribution to a set of ongoing and exciting research programs.

NOTES

1. The Conference was held at the University of Pittsburgh in 1978. Papers were assembled over the following three years, and several have been revised as recently as 1983.

2. See especially Hanson 1958, 1961.

3. A good historical account of these developments in philosophy of science can be found in the lengthy introduction to Suppe 1977.

4. See Nickles 1980 for papers from a national conference on the logic of scientific discovery. Also see Nickles, in press, for an account of some of the recent developments in this area.

5. See Szolovits and Pauker 1978, Schaffner 1981, and Pople 1982 for discussion and references on this topic.

6. See Schaffner 1980 for a discussion of the contexts of discovery and justification and for references to the historical-philosophical literature.

7. See Feinstein 1969, 451. A more developed analysis of the logic of diagnosis can be found in Feinstein 1973–1974.

8. For some important criticisms of the Bayesian approach to diagnosis see Szolovits and Pauker 1978 and also the references in Schaffner 1981.

9. See Miller, Pople, and Myers 1982 as well as Schaffner 1981.

10. See Schaffner 1981, 165 for discussion and references.

11. As noted below in the text, these values are judgmental; they can change and from time to time have changed somewhat. The present values are taken from Miller, Pople, and Myers 1982; for an earlier set of values see Schaffner 1981, 187 n. 9, and McMullin's essay in this volume.

12. A pathognomonic manifestation is one of those rare findings in medicine which taken alone would permit the observer to conclude immediately a specific diagnosis; i.e., it is logically sufficient for that diagnosis. An example might be the Kayser-Fleisher ring seen in the cornea in Wilson's syndrome. Interestingly, in an earlier INTERNIST-I scoring scheme the program concluded when the spread was 80 rather than 90 points. This, however, led to too many unwarranted diagnoses.

13. I think this point is arguable. My position is based on the fact that factoring in such a heuristic could well lead to premature diagnostic closure and thus to serious errors of not diagnosing a disease that was in fact treatable because the patient's problem was not pursued far enough.

14. In addition, it was soon realized that a "multistep synthesis operator" permitting a "jump" over an intervening node whose status is unknown would be needed.

15. See Schaffner 1980 for parallels between INTERNIST-I's stages and the processes followed by MacFarlane Burnet in his discovery of the clonal-selection theory of the immune response.

REFERENCES

Bobrow, R. H., and J. S. Brown. 1975. Systematic understanding: Synthesis, analysis and contingent knowledge in specialized understanding systems.

In *Representation and understanding,* ed. D. Bobrow and A. Collins. New York: Academic Press.

Buchanan, B. G. 1985. Steps toward mechanizing discovery. In this volume.

Clouser, K. D. 1985. Approaching the logic of diagnosis. In this volume.

Engelhardt, H. T. 1985. Typologies of disease: Nosologies revisited. In this volume.

Feinstein, A. 1969. Taxonomy and logic in clinical data. *Annals of the New York Academy of Science* 161:450–459.

———. 1973–74. An analysis of diagnostic reasoning. *Yale Journal of Biology and Medicine* 46:212–232, 264–283; 47:5–32.

Hanson, N. R. 1958. *Patterns of discovery.* Cambridge: Cambridge University Press.

———. 1961. Is there a logic of discovery? In *Current issues in the philosophy of science,* ed. H. Feigl and G. Maxwell, 20–42. New York: Holt, Rinehart & Winston.

Hempel, C. G. 1985. Thoughts on the limitations of discovery by computer. In this volume.

Holland, J. 1975. *Adaptation in natural and artificial systems.* Ann Arbor: University of Michigan Press.

———. 1980. Adaptive algorithms for discovering and using general patterns in growing knowledge bases. *Journal of Policy Analysis and Information Systems* 4:217–240.

Kyburg, H. E. 1985. The logic(s) of evaluation in basic and clinical science. In this volume.

Lenat, D. 1977. The ubiquity of discovery. *Artificial Intelligence* 9:257–285.

McMullin, E. 1985. Diagnosis by computer. In this volume.

Miller, R. A., H. E. Pople, and J. D. Myers. 1982. INTERNIST-I, an experimental computer-based diagnostic consultant for general internal medicine. *New England Journal of Medicine* 307:468–476.

Myers, J. D. 1985. The process of clinical diagnosis and its adaptation to the computer. In this volume.

Newell, A., J. C. Shaw, and H. Simon. [1962] 1979. The processes of creative thinking. Reprinted in *Models of thought,* ed. H. Simon, 144–174. New Haven: Yale University Press.

Newell, A., and H. Simon. 1972. *Human problem solving.* Englewood Cliffs, N.J.: Prentice-Hall.

Nickles, T., ed. 1980. *Scientific discovery, logic, and rationality.* 2 vols. Dordrecht: Reidel.

———. In press. Beyond the divorce thesis: Current status of the discovery debate. Circulated draft version, 28 Sept. 1983.

Nilsson, N. J. 1980. *Principles of artificial intelligence.* Palo Alto, Calif.: Tioga.

Nugent, C. A., et al. 1964. Probability theory in diagnosis of Cushing's syndrome. *Journal of Clinical Endocrinology* 24:621–627.

Patil, R., P. Szolovits, and W. B. Schwartz. 1981. Causal understanding of patient illness in medical diagnosis. In *Proceedings of the Seventh International Joint Conference on Artificial Intelligence*, 892–899.

Polya, G. 1957. *How to solve it.* Princeton: Princeton University Press.

Pople, H. E. 1982. Heuristic methods for imposing structure on ill-structured problems: The structuring of medical diagnostics. In *Artificial intelligence in medicine*, 119–185. See Szolovits 1982.

———. 1985. Coming to grips with the multiple-diagnosis problem. In this volume.

Schaffner, K. F. 1980. Discovery in the biomedical sciences: Logic or irrational intuition? In *Scientific discovery, logic and rationality* 2:171–205. See Nickles 1980.

———. 1981. Modeling medical diagnosis: Logical and computer approaches. *Synthese* 47:163–199.

Seidenfeld, T. 1985. More on the logic(s) of evaluation in basic and clinical science. In this volume.

Simon, H. 1977. *Models of discovery.* Dordrecht: Reidel.

———. 1985. Artificial-intelligence approaches to problem solving and clinical diagnosis. In this volume.

Simon, H., P. Langley, and G. L. Bradshaw. 1981. Scientific discovery as problem solving. *Synthese* 47:1–27.

Suppe, F., ed. 1977. *The structure of scientific theories.* 2d. ed. Champaign-Urbana: University of Illinois Press.

Szolovits, P., ed. 1982. *Artificial intelligence in medicine.* Boulder, Colo.: Westview Press.

Szolovits, P., and S. Pauker. 1978. Categorical and probabalistic reasoning in medical diagnosis. *Artificial Intelligence* 11:115–144.

Weiss, S. M., C. A. Kulikowski, S. Amarel, and A. Safir. 1978. A model-based method for computer-aided medical decision-making. *Artificial Intelligence* 11:145–172.

Whitbeck, C. 1981. What is diagnosis? A preface to the investigation of clinical reasoning. *Metamedicine* 2:319–329.

Wulff, H. R. 1976. *Rational diagnosis and treatment.* Oxford: Blackwell.

———. 1981. *Rational diagnosis and treatment.* 2d. ed. Oxford: Blackwell.

PART ONE
General Considerations

1

Approaching the Logic
of Diagnosis

K. Danner Clouser

INTRODUCTION

We have all had the experience of attending a conference in our own
or a related speciality and being hit cold with a tidal wave of
technicalities. From the first word following the welcome, we are torn
from our customary moorings and tossed hither and yon by waves of
speakers. We get fleeting glimpses of familiar landmarks, but never
enough, nor for long enough, to get our bearings.

It is the assigned role of this paper to be a kind of footbath, a wading
pool, before the plunge. Its job as footbath is to warm the reader up,
to get him acclimated, and by all means, to remain shallow.

This paper will approach diagnosis very broadly and very gently.
While gradually immersing the reader in the topic, it will faintly focus
attention on certain areas, so that the *real* articles that follow may be
read more expectantly and searchingly.

My aim will be to write as though I were talking both to practicing
physicians who are mildly surprised to hear others referring to a
"logic" of diagnosis (always having themselves believed it was more
of an art, intuition, or just good sense) and to philosophers who always
thought diagnosis was simply following a recipe of sorts. Perhaps no

such naive doctors and philosophers even exist, but the concept of such provides an imaginable group of people toward whom these introductory comments may be directed. These comments may well be far beneath most readers—but that's what footbaths are all about.

My plan is to mention and very briefly describe the variety of recent interests in medical decision-making and the variety of uses to which computers have been put in the medical context. Then I will close in on the process of diagnosis, isolating some of its elements and describing in a general way some strategies at work there. For the second half of the paper, as a means of drawing out certain aspects of diagnosis for a slightly closer look, I will consider some obvious contributions a computer could make and will give voice to some initial worries a practicing clinician might well have about computer diagnosis.

APPROACHES TO DIAGNOSTIC REASONING: AN OVERVIEW

It might be worthwhile for an overall perspective to have a thumbnail description of research that has been going on with some intensity since the 1950s. The struggle to organize medical information has been one of the major problems in contemporary medical research.[1]

One can crudely distinguish two general emphases or directions to the research. The first is the attempt to understand the human cognitive processes at work in problem solving. The other is the development of computer programs for doing a variety of jobs in handling considerable amounts of data. The two, of course, are not unrelated. The delving into human problem-solving processes was really an effort to describe the logic of the process, the sequence of steps, the management and weighting of variables, and other such strategies. The hope was to abstract the formulas, algorithms, decision rules, or whatever could accurately replicate the human problem-solver at work. This could be used to improve human reasoning, to teach it to others, or to provide clues and insights for constructing computer programs.

The analysis of human problem-solving processes takes many different and ingenious forms.[2] Attempting to capture and describe human thought-processes is an elusive enterprise. Whether researchers are abstracting from what the expert diagnostician (as experimental subject in this case) has written on paper or spoken into a dictaphone, or whether they are pressing him to introspect each step of the way, we cannot help but wonder if the researchers' foci, questions, and task descriptions have interfered with the very reasoning process they are trying to observe. Yet with their results they are able to replicate fairly accurately the expert clinician's judgments. And though that does not mean they have accurately described the processes themselves, the results have been interesting and helpful. It seems clear, for example, that experts ask fewer questions and get the maximum yield from each question.[3] It also appears that experts in making judgments use far fewer variables than they themselves had thought they were using and that they are not giving the variables the differential weighting they thought they were.[4] And so the analysis goes, not only describing the efficient processes of the best problem-solvers but finding wherein there may be some built-in biases, such as failing to update one's data bank even though one has the information to do so, giving equal weight to all information by disregarding its relative strengths, weaknesses, sources, certainty, and so on, tending to construe data on the simplest relevant model, and remembering only positive correlations and not negative ones.[5] Like analyzing the hook in one's golf swing, these are partly efforts to alert clinicians to their strengths and biases in hopes of improving performance.

Paralleling the research into the cognitive processes of diagnosis, there have been other branches of research in organizing medical information—the use of computers.

The strength of computers is obviously that they can handle massive amounts of information, and with incredible speed. There are a variety of mathematic models and modes of logic incorporated in the variety of computers at work.[6] Some of the complexities of these will be dealt with in subsequent articles. These "logics" each have their strengths, their drawbacks, and their special facility for certain tasks. Many computers are programmed to handle a particular diagnostic or therapeutic problem, such as with cardiovascular maladies,[7] antimicrobial therapy,[8] or electrolyte and acid-base disorders.[9] In this role the computer asks further questions, leads the physician to more specific categorizations, suggests more decisive tests, and even offers appropriate bibliographical references. It is acting like a consultant. In this use the computer is an extension of the physician—enlarging his memory, his data bank, and sharpening his line of reasoning and his differential diagnosis. Speed also can be an extremely important factor, as in the case of myocardial infarct or in figuring a therapeutic dosage for a patient in a diabetic coma.[10] When many variables must be considered, when there exist dozens of subgroups within a disease classification, each of which needs different immediate therapy for the best chances of survival, when a speedy diagnosis is essential, computers are exceptionally helpful.

Other computers are designed more for pattern recognition and so for such tasks as reading chest X rays[11] and serial electrocardiograms.[12] Still others are "on-line" computers connected to the patient, giving immediate feedback, correlations, and next-step guidance instantaneously with the measurement of the data. This has been done with electrocardiograms, with heart auscultation, and with human-metabolism data.[13] Computers can be used for general screening purposes as has been done for heretofore unrecognized diabetes mellitus.[14]

And finally, computers have been used in teaching differential diagnosis[15] and in the management of patients in connection with a patient-oriented computer-based medical record.[16]

The only point of the foregoing impressionistic thumbnail description of research in medical decision-making in the last decade or so is simply to heighten our awareness that there has been considerable activity and, as one might guess, a complexity commensurate with such activity.

ELEMENTS OF DIAGNOSIS:
A WHIMSICAL WARM-UP

We come now to the central part of this inaugural paper's task, which is to start us thinking more specifically and as gently as possible about medical diagnosis. These observations will be articulated for those clinicians and philosophers who have never reflected on the reasoning process itself or on the logic of medical diagnosis. Even though there may be no such person, the purpose of a gentle warm-up is nevertheless served. Even accomplished athletes begin each performance with the same trivial calisthenics the rest of us do.

In working up a patient, physicians are blending at least two activities: one is the gathering of information, and the other is the attempt to see a pattern or a constellation in those data. It is the pattern-seeing that might more technically be called the diagnosis. The physician is wanting to put the patient in a classification because the physician's knowledge of causes, treatment, and prognoses is organized that way. In trying to arrive at a classification, that is, a disease or illness label, the processes of data gathering and diagnosis are in no set sequence. The physician goes back and forth; progress on one front gives rise to suggested possibilities on the other. For example, upon simply looking at a patient, a physician might immediately entertain a probable diagnosis (i.e., a hypothesis), and that in turn would suggest some data to be gathered to confirm or disconfirm the probable diagnosis. This is to assert something that philosophers have known (one way or another) for a long time, namely, that those introductory chapters of science textbooks describing the so-called "scientific method" had to be all wrong. Such books would have us believe that we first gather all the facts and then we formulate our hypotheses . . . and so on. But of course our hypotheses, or initial guesses, are instrumental in suggesting which of the infinite facts surrounding us should be attended to, and this seems especially true of medical diagnosis.

When a physician is presented with a patient, one major factor in his reasoning may not be consciously entertained at all, yet it surely plays a critical role. The physician is aware of likelihoods of certain sicknesses among the people who generally consult him. He by no means regards every conceivable disease as equally likely. His mindset, as it were, is influenced by what he generally sees, and that is determined by whether he is a referral physician, whether he practices in a hot or a cold climate, whether he is in a culture without food refrigeration, and so on for hundreds of variables. In short, the strength of a physician's initial disposition to regard his patient as having a certain illness is directly proportional to the incidence of that disease in the population he serves. (That isn't quite true, of course, but it will do for now.) As the old cliché has it, upon hearing hoofbeats in the distance we should not anticipate zebras (unless of course they are very, very distant!). What we are talking about is technically called "prior probability," and in our current context it refers to the incidence in the population of the disease in question. If the flu bug is on a rampage, and your patient presents with fever and chills, the prior probability that your patient has the flu is quite high, although of course it could conceivably turn out to be tuberculosis or malaria.

To ignore prior probability in confronting a patient is equivalent to regarding every disease as equally probable. To be sure, this would significantly increase one's chance of detecting the rarer diseases, but it would also mean that the diagnostician would have to start from scratch on each case. Taking prior probability into account gives one a good working hypothesis to start from, temporarily ruling out many, many other possibilities. Prior probability also makes a significant difference in the predictive value of test results, as we shall see (cf. note 27).

A diagnostician friend of mine insists on sending patients to the radiologist and tissues to the pathologist without *any* accompanying information about the patient concerned. For the radiologist or pathologist, that is like trying to understand a spoken syllable with no other verbal context, or in the wrong verbal context. For X rays or tissues, it is seldom a black-and-white matter. It is ambiguous, and experts can disagree—even with their own earlier interpretation. And if they are not even told some of the physical signs and symptoms, they cannot narrow down the population with which they are dealing. If they cannot define their population to get a prior probability estimate, their estimate of the test result would be considerably off, as we shall see in more detail later. Ideally they would know the odds of this patient's having the disease without even looking at the X rays or tissue, and then, having the test results, would further refine that probability. In short, the value of the tests should be in how much beyond the prior probability they will take him.

We turn now to the heart of any diagnostic reasoning: the relationship between signs, symptoms, lab tests, and so on, and the disease of which they are manifestations. We need not be concerned with causal relationships but only with sheer correlations. What can the presence of the one tell us about the possible presence of the other, statistically? That is, given the one, what is the probability of the other's being there? Given the disease, what is the probability of having such and such a symptom? Or, what is more often the question in a diagnostic context, given the symptom, what is the probability of having such and such a disease? (For convenience I will mean by *symptom* any manifestation, sign, test, or behavior.) The physician no doubt has a rough notion of what the likelihood is of having the symptom, given the disease. That is, from past experience, or from medical records, or from the literature, one might find out how many instances of a particular disease were accompanied by a certain symptom. Perhaps seven out of every ten patients with TB had hemoptysis (i.e., spitting up blood). So, given that the patient has the disease, the probability of his having the symptom of hemoptysis is .7. But remember, what we usually want to know in diagnosis is the probability of the patient's having this or that disease, given the symptoms he is manifesting. This is just the converse of what we might find out from records or the literature, namely, given the disease, what is the incidence of the symptom. In the diagnostic context, the physician is given the symptom, and is trying to figure out the probability of this or that disease in his patient, given the symptom. Impressionistically, then, if there is a high prior probability (i.e., a high incidence of the disease in the population) and if most people with the disease have the symptom in question, then the probability of this particular patient's having the disease seems quite high. If, however, the prior probability or the probability of the symptom (given the disease) or both were lower, so also would the probability that the patient has the disease be lower.

But, just a minute! No matter how many diseased people have this symptom, if lots of other people also have the same symptom and they are either well or have some *other* disease, then the probability that our symptomatic patient has the disease in question is considerably reduced. In other words, if a lot of people have the symptom—say, a rapid heartbeat—who do not have the disease in question, then the chances that a patient who presents with a rapid heartbeat has that disease are lessened a good bit.

So far we have interrelated three factors in our impressionistic diagnosis: the incidence of the suspected disease in the population overall, multiplied by the odds (established from past experience) of patients' having this symptom if they have the disease. That product would give us the likelihood of our symptomatic patient's having the disease. But this likelihood is further reduced by the proportion of the people in this same population who also have the symptom but who do *not* have that disease.

It would be well to stop at this point for some commentary about and around what we have been doing.

1. Many readers by now recognize a gross form of Bayes' theorem emerging. I am not suggesting that a systematic calculation of probabilities is going on in a diagnostician's mind, but I am suggesting that these are some major factors entering into a clinician's reasoning. No doubt he is subjectively (and probably erratically) estimating the likelihoods and intuitively combining them to arrive at his degree of certainty about the presence of

a particular disease in his patient. (Obviously this account is more normative than descriptive. Only those empirical psychologists tracing the process of diagnostic reasoning are to be trusted with what *actually* is being thought by their sampling of expert diagnosticians.)

2. A wild guess as to why the old general practitioner was so often right (besting the specialists on some occasions in my experience) is that he really knew his prior probabilities. He knew the incidence of that disease in his population; and he knew the incidence of symptoms that existed independently of that disease. A child's strange behavior might lead a neurologist to be sure the child had a bad disease, because one out of every three who came to see him with that symptom had such a disease. The old G.P. might have said, "Heck, my office is full of kids that act that way, and they aren't sick." Without realizing it, he knew his prior probabilities, and he was also, without realizing it, intuitively doing statistics.

3. None of this will be making sense if one has the wrong notion about the pattern of relationships between and among symptoms and their diseases. It is in fact less like matching samples to a master color chart and more like looking into a kaleidoscope.

   Maladies are not neat packages with their very own characteristic markings. As they get expressed in each individual human, they can look quite diverse. The uniqueness of each human—right down to his genes and proteins—makes a unique context within which any particular malady interacts and manifests itself. Then add to that mixture the laboratory findings that can be influenced by lab error, by daily fluctuations of the patient or of the lab technician or of the pathologist, by the unrepresentative specimen that happened to have been obtained, by the sensitivity or specificity of the tests, and so on. A so-called "textbook" or "classic" case is exciting precisely because it does not come along all that often! It is in this context of cascading variables that we recognize why statistical methods—intuitive or explicit—seem necessary. Only statistics seem able to handle the high degree of variability and the complex pattern of correlated data. With so many variables, practically nothing comes clear and distinct; there are thousands of combinations possible. So calculating the odds of this and that, given such and such, seems the only way to have a reasonable basis for decisions.

What we have done so far in examining diagnosis is, of course, qualitative and terribly oversimplified. We have looked at statistical relationships between a symptom and its disease, seeing what increases and what diminishes the probability of one, given the other. In the real world there would be many symptoms and signs and test results with varying probabilities (alone or in combination) of being indicative of one or another disease. But more about that later.

We notably have not been considering the overall organization or sequence of reasoning. After all, a patient is not the probability theorist's bag of black and white marbles whose total composition the physician estimates inductively from the symptom sample described by the patient. Some symptoms the patient will have observed, others the physician must elicit, and still other conditions await studies and tests to uncover their presence. There are thousands of questions and thousands of tests. Can there possibly be an order to them? Is there a sequence that is more fruitful than most? Is there a way to keep from going down too many blind alleys?

Many have thought there to be a kind of branching logic at work. It is generally a binomial system, that is, a simple yes or no to each question, with follow-up questions branching from each of those answers, and so on. But it would seem awfully easy to bark up (or down) the wrong decision tree, unless (1) the sequence of questions is just right and (2) all the contingencies are specified in advance.[17] If the diagnostician began with several not very discriminating questions, he would be quickly branching out in the wrong direction. But this branching is helpful when initial conditions have significantly limited the area to be explored. Perhaps one is trying to differentiate this illness from several that look very much like it, or perhaps the genus malady is clear and one is trying to find what subclassification the instant case falls into. And, in fact, I suspect the branching logic is the most frequently used process, precisely because initial conditions (such as previous acquaintance with the patient, the prior probability of a given illness with the presenting symptoms, the symptoms reported by the patient himself) and especially the history and physical are sufficient for the diagnostician to leap rapidly to a hypothesis, which he proceeds to confirm or disconfirm. (And as we saw earlier, the empirical researchers tracing mental processes of clinicians say the clinicians move very directly and quickly to an array of provisional hypotheses.)[18]

Having a hypothesis in mind, he can pursue a line of yes/no questions that certainly branch, but in a restricted area, where one at least cannot go far astray. Nevertheless, sequence of questions is important, if only to save time. For example, in dealing with a neurological disorder one might pursue many questions attempting to find the rough location of a tumor, though there might have been a prior question (say, whether it was a symmetrical syndrome or an acute onset) that would have ruled out a tumor much earlier. (It has been pointed out that experienced diagnosticians get the diagnosis quicker and with fewer questions, all of which are more discriminatory, and, one would think, in the most economic sequence.)[19]

But we should remember that hypothesis testing is simply a way of *using* the statistical relations between symptom and disease which we discussed earlier. That is, a yes or no answer to a branching question almost never categorically places a case into a specific disease group or subgroup; rather, given that yes or no (with respect to the positive finding of a particular symptom, sign, or test result), there is only a certain probability that this case falls into one group or another, and that probability is enhanced or diminished by those factors we discussed earlier.

The last factor in diagnosis to be highlighted in our cursory glimpse is the matter of values.

Whether or not values enter into the "logic" of diagnosis depends on how wide one's conception of logic is. Some might think of logic as precisely that which excludes values. But if "logic" is thought of as the formal, systematic procedures for drawing inferences and conclusions, then explicit attention to values is probably in order. Very generally, when conclusions must be acted upon and probabilities are all we have to go on, then we have no alternative but to weigh carefully the value of what we have to win or lose against the odds of winning or losing. For example, in some situations, there being not much to lose and something to be gained, we will go with lower odds; if a lot might be lost if we are wrong, we want higher probabilities that we are right before we act. Some might argue that values do not enter diagnosis per se, but only more broadly into "clinical judgment." I will not argue the point here but will be content with observing that if deciding what tests to order involves value judgments, and if tests are essential aspects of diagnosis, then values come very close indeed to diagnosis.

Values come into play because we are considering actions that affect people, and these actions are based on something considerably less than certainty. For example, consider the relevant factors in the simple and frequent questions of whether or not to run further tests on a patient. How sure are we of our diagnosis with the test? How accurate are the tests? How expensive, painful, frightening, or time-consuming are the tests? What might be lost if we began therapy for what we suspect without doing the further tests? On the other hand, what risks are we running if we skip the tests and do not do any therapy? Is it a risk worth taking? From whose point of view? Is there a risk of the disease spreading to other people? Add these personal valuings and weightings to the subjective estimates of all the probabilities involved, and one quickly understands the need for systematizing and even computerizing diagnosis.

Some have suggested that we build decision trees for therapy decisions.[20] Each branch has a probability figure, so that one can see at a glance all the different possible outcomes of the patient before us, depending on all the various therapy actions that might be taken along the height and the width of the decision tree. This requires listing all the possible outcomes and the probability of each one's coming to pass. Then the vigorously blossoming tree is trimmed by sawing off those branches which fall below some arbitrarily drawn level of probability. Presumably something like a decision tree is always going on in the physician's mind—much as when pondering our next move in a chess game, we play out as best we can in our minds the evolving sequence of moves and countermoves for each possibility we are entertaining. Building the tree explicitly on paper or with a computer is simply being much more accurate.

We do not have time to look into each avenue of value-ladenness in diagnosis and therapy in detail, so we will take only one as an example; it is old hat to physicians, but perhaps not to philosophers. This is the matter of the "sensitivity" and "specificity" of diagnostic tests. Defining those terms here would create confusion beyond necessity. It is sufficient to say that almost all diagnostic tests produce some false positives (i.e., the test indicates the patient has the disease in question when in fact the patient does not have the disease) and some false negatives (i.e., the test indicates the patient does not have the disease, when in fact the patient does have the disease). The percentages of each can usually be determined, and the physician can enter those probabilities into his calculations. For example, he might figure that even though the test indicates the presence of disease in his patient, there is nevertheless a, say, 10% chance of the test being wrong.

There are value decisions at two levels: the first in the laboratory and the second in the doctor's office. The one in the laboratory concerns where the line is drawn dividing the negatives from the positives. That is, suppose the presence of a disease is correlated with an increased amount of some substance X in the blood. Now at the two extremes where there is no X in the blood and where there is a maximum amount of X in the blood, we can be sure that there is *no* disease at the low end and that there *is* disease at the high end of this continuous range. A large section somewhere in the center will be ambiguous; some people with those amounts of X will have the disease, and some with the same amounts will not. If we shift the dividing line toward the high end of the scale, we will be increasing the number of false negatives (i.e., we will be telling more people they do not have the disease, when in fact they do). If we shift the dividing line toward the low end of the scale, we will increase the number of false positives (i.e., we will be telling more people they have the disease, when in fact they do not). Among the factors to be considered in drawing the line is the cost of misdiagnosis in both directions. What is the cost, in terms of pain, loss of life, expense, delay of treatment, worry, contagion, and so on, of labeling a condition a disease when it is not, versus labeling it free of disease when in fact disease is present?

In the office there are parallels with the laboratory's line drawing that demarcates false negatives and false positives. The physician is not drawing the line, but he is interpreting the results of that line's having been drawn. Knowing the probability of false negatives and false positives of a given diagnostic test, he must weigh the statistics of the other symptoms and signs of his patient and decide the cost of misdiagnosis. One could even assign numerical values to figure in with the probabilities of the various diagnoses. Suppose, for example, the physician were trying to differentiate several possible disease states of his patient: a simple goiter, Hashimoto's disease, and carcinoma of the thyroid.[21] Without introducing details, one can intuitively see that there would be ways of assigning relative weights to these in order to minimize the chances of misdiagnosing a more serious disease as a nonserious disease. Thus, the high probability of the simple goiter would be mathematically diminished by the assigned value, and the slight probability of the carcinoma would be heightened by the assigned numerical value, proportionately to the seriousness of misclassifying it as something less risky. Needless to say, the assignment of these relative weightings should raise many questions. However, that line of analysis is perhaps more appropriate for the field of ethics.

COULD A COMPUTER HELP?

We have now completed our simplified overview of the diagnostic process, highlighting factors influencing the conclusions drawn—that is, loosely speaking, the "logic" of diagnosis.

Now, as a method of securing some of the previous points, we will ask two questions on a very general level: Can computers help? And what worries might one have (at least initially) about computer diagnosis? It must be emphasized that this is not meant to be a help to computer diagnosticians; they are already far beyond this level. Rather it is simply a pedagogical means of turning our thoughts to more details concerning the logic of diagnosis.

The simple and obvious answer to the first question is, "Of course." A computer could be of enormous help to a diagnostician, if only in complementing his work. The enormous data bank necessary for accurate probabilities, the encyclopedic and essential information about diseases, symptoms, and therapies, far surpass the amount a person's mind can retain.

Somewhat more specifically, many researchers have reported fascinating things about man as a decision maker.[22] He is good at making subjective estimates of probabilities but very bad at combining them; he is very conservative in his estimates, failing to take into account new data, yet generally seeking more information than is necessary; he tends to remember only positive correlations and not negative ones; and he tends to be skewed in his probabilistic judgments by recent and dramatic cases.[23] All these apparently natural inclinations could be overcome by the neutral accuracy of a computer, noted for its nonsubjective, nonerratic, nonimpresssionable, nonforgetful behavior. For example, the prior probability (i.e., the incidence of the disease in question in the general population) enormously influences a physician's estimation of the case before him.[24] Yet his own estimate of this is notoriously subjective and biased. A computer could be not only accurate, but constantly and instantly up to date, as each new case was recorded. The same could be true of those probability relations between symptom and diagnosis. We also know that humans can handle only a very limited amount of information in their heads and that in estimating probability they are more apt to rely on rules of thumb than on frequency.[25]

These same calculation difficulties would also apply to the quantification of values, as we saw earlier. We currently do this very impressionistically. There may be an important virtue in having to make these values explicit and precise enough to enter into the equations being handled by the computer.

These meandering and obvious observations of computer helpfulness will cease after one more example. We have seen how the diagnostic process deals with many probabilities and usually does so intuitively. But these can be far off base in a dangerous way. Suppose there is a population of 1,000 people, and there is a prior probability for a given disease of 1% (i.e., 1% of that population actually has the disease). Furthermore, suppose the relevant diagnostic test has a sensitivity of 95% (i.e., 95 out of every 100 persons with the disease will have a positive test result) and a specificity of 95% (i.e., 95 out of 100 persons without the disease will have negative test results). Your patient has a positive test result. What is the likelihood (based only on that test) that he has the disease? Apparently, many or most physicians in similar estimations would place the odds very high.[26] Actually, in this case there is only a 16% chance that your patient has the disease.[27] This one example simply reminds us how important the prior probability is and how far off our intuitive guesses of probabilities might be. A crucial factor for the predictive value of a positive test is the incidence of the disease in the population; that is what we have been calling "prior probability." Roughly, the higher the prior probability, the higher the predictive value of a positive test. For such reasons, defining populations and updating disease incidence are of great importance. Presumably a computer could help us to be considerably more accurate and might even help us to recalibrate our intuitions (though admittedly, in this particular example, pencil and paper would no doubt be sufficient!).

COMPUTERIZING DIAGNOSIS:
SOME CONCERNS

These may not be important concerns, but they constitute an attempt to give voice to the first thoughts of novices. As mentioned earlier, the diagnostic computerists are way ahead of us in subtleties and solutions. But as a means of drawing our attention to interesting conceptual items within diagnosis and thereby warming us up for the subsequent papers, this "list of concerns" is as fruitful a tactic as any.

The questioning begins appropriately with the notion of prior probability. The central problem is one of defining or designating the population whose incidence of a given disease is in question. Is it a certain age group? Obviously, for some diseases the incidence of disease would be very different from that of the population at large. Do we determine the incidence by the group of those persons who populate the health care facilities? If so, surely the incidence of given diseases would vary greatly from subgroup to subgroup: those who come to a family physician, those who come to the emergency room, those who come to see specialists, and so on. Furthermore, geographic differences, weather differences, and seasonal differences change the incidence of one or another illness. So individuating the population is a critical issue since, as we have seen, it greatly influences our guess as to what the particular patient before us has, and consequently our decision on how to manage him, and it greatly influences the percentage of false positives and false negatives we might expect. The reason this might become even more problematic with a computer is that everyone serving different populations might be feeding disease statistics into it, whereas now the ordinary clinician no doubt simply makes a subjective estimate on the basis of those he usually sees. And perhaps the latter is more apt to be accurate for diagnostic reasoning purposes than the widely pooled information.

A second but related problem is the matter of differing stages of disease. As symptoms of a particular disease become more pronounced, or recede, or new ones replace old ones, the probability relationships between symptom and disease become clouded and considerably less useful. Perhaps for both prior probability and symptom/disease conditional probability we will have to specify the *stage* of the disease in question. This will complicate calculations enormously, since that, in effect, is like increasing the number of diseases to be dealt with four- or fivefold! And it is possible that we already have more units of information and combinations than the computer can handle.[28]

Further related to these complications of prior probability and conditional probabilities is the problem of multiple diseases. Are we dealing with a mildly unusual version of one disease, or actually with two or three overlapping diseases? Must we logically treat each possible combination of diseases as itself a disease, in which case we again make the number of diseases unmanageable? At the very least we (or the computer) must keep careful track of which symptoms are being accounted for in our proposed diagnosis, and which are left over, unexplained. For Bayes' theorem to work accurately, there must be the assumption that all the diseases are mutually exclusive and that the sum of their probabilities is one. Yet that obviously is not the case. However, there may already be so much slack in estimating prior probabilities that this additional wrinkle will not be noticed![29]

Perhaps the knottiest problem of all has to do with the so-called "assumption of independence" necessary in Bayes' theorem. This is a complicated matter and is raised here only to convey an intuitive notion of the issue.

We have been talking simplistically of the conditional probability of a particular symptom given a particular disease. The assumption has been that the likelihood of that symptom's occurring with that disease is completely independent of some other symptom's occurring with that disease. The effect of this is to bias the probability calculations against two or more symptoms occurring together. But in fact they almost always do. For example, the likelihood that symptom X occurs with a particular disease might be high; consequently the presence of that symptom suggests a high probability that our patient has the disease. But there may be another symptom Y that also has a high likelihood of concurrence with that disease. But when combined by multiplication they *reduce* the probability that our patient has the disease, when intuitively we would think that the occurrence of both symptoms would serve to enhance the probability that our patient has the disease. By treating the symptoms as independent occurrences, we, in effect, make it a remarkable event (i.e., a less probable event), a coincidence, that they should appear together—like the odds of two or three lemons lining up in a slot-machine window. But in fact, these symptoms are seldom independent ontologically. They are causally connected in the patient, or, if not with each other, perhaps with some third thing. Indeed, it is not infrequently the case that each of two symptoms independently has only a very low correlation with a disease state but that the two taken together have a high correlation and hence discriminatory power.

Consequently, one would guess that probabilities would be far more powerful if we considered the probability of various combinations of symptoms, given the disease. But it does not take much imagination to see the exponential rise in the number of factors and probabilities to be handled. If we had n symptoms to keep track of before, we would now have 2^n—and that assumes only the (binary) combinations of *pairs.* The mere twenty symptoms that we might have kept track of on the assumption of independence would now become 1,048,576 possible combinations.[30]

There have been a variety of very complicated ways proposed to deal with the matter of dependent symptoms. The essence of them seems to be this: Do analysis to find which pairs or clusters of symptoms are most frequent or most discriminatory or most closely biologically linked, and then, in figuring probabilities, treat that "unit" as if it were an independent symptom correlated with the disease state in question.

We dealt with the values issue earlier. No more analysis of that is to the point here, but in light of what we have already done, a quick observation with respect to computer diagnosis is worth making. We saw how value weighting was possible and why it was necessary. The problem is that there are many values such as cost, pain, inconvenience, worry, and permanent complications to be weighed, and they all get reduced to one numerical value that functions as the so-called "utility factor." As good as it is to have the place and weight of value in these considerations isolated and examined explicitly, nevertheless, transmuting these diverse golden rays into a single lead weight is conceivably worse than not imagining that one has accounted for values at all. A case in point is the health index used as the quantitative measure of success for various modes of therapy. In combining mortality and morbidity into a single index (though a vast improvement over sheer economic considerations), there is allowed a trade-off between length of life and quality of life, such that success (or health improvement) is proved for a drug or mode of therapy if longevity increases, even though the misery of that life is intense.[31]

At long last, the final issue for our attention is what might be roughly thought of as "the art of medicine." No attempt will be made to explicate that notion here.[32] But simply in its ordinary sense (though specifically excluding bedside manner), one might wonder if any of it would be lost in computer diagnosis. Are the clinical intuitions and sensitivities still crucial to pick up clues that would otherwise be missed and for which there seem to be no rules, no heuristics, no algorithms? Of course, if we could say what kind of items this intuition picked up, if we could describe the process, if we could say what more it is than the steps and procedures of problem solving and decision making, then we could in fact build it into the computer. Perhaps it is nothing more; perhaps it is just that our "reduction" of diagnosis and problem solving is not yet complete.

One might worry that as computers are more and more used for diagnosis, the operator will more and more lose his sensitivities to all the nuances, the problematic, the borderline, the multiplicity of values (reduced no doubt to a single number), and will simply put total faith in the readout; he will become a technician whose world slowly but inexorably becomes increasingly black and white. Yet we are mindful that even now a totally human diagnostician frequently says that such and such "is medically indicated," suggesting a hard-and-fast and unarguable "readout," even though we know that all kinds of subjective probabilities and value deliberations went into that decision, which is now posing as a rigorous scientific deduction.

One need not be a mystical intuitionist to argue that, so far, at least, it seems that formalisms alone will not lead to what could be described as intelligent behavior. A clinician gains understanding and clues from a patient's choice of words, his facial expressions, his gestures, his movements, and his subliminal messages. The clinician can empathize with the patient's emotional state and come to see how the patient is interpreting his illness. Nevertheless, our constant attempt to unpack our intelligent behavior and to reproduce it in the formalisms of various logics is probably the best route to the progressive discovery, refinement, and computer imitation of those elusive human qualities (though some argue that in principle it is impossible ever to achieve).[33]

In so many of the computer-diagnosis programs, one cannot help being struck by the role of the human physician as intermediary between the patient and the machine. The trained eye still does the initial appraising, the overall evaluating (the assessment of the presenting symptoms, the look of the patient, the subjective estimate of the prior probabilities), the physical exam, and usually the history. The physician is thus the funnel through which all this cornucopia of variables is narrowed down to a manageable area of investigation that is then taken over by computer. A happy compromise, according to some, would be to say that humans are ideal for acquisition of the facts and computers are ideal for performing the actuarial methods used to deal with those facts. It would seem, however, that the eliciting of facts cannot be distinguished all that clearly from the processing of and reasoning by means of those facts. But that, the reader should be relieved to learn, is another story.

NOTES

1. L. B. Lusted, *Introduction to Medical Decision Making* (Springfield, Ill.: Charles C Thomas, 1968).

2. The most recent work is A. Elstein, L. Shulman, and S. Sprafka, *Medical Problem Solving: An Analysis of Clinical Reasoning* (Cambridge: Harvard Univ. Press, 1978). Chap. 2 (pp. 10–45) comprises an excellent recent history of the various efforts to analyze clinical reasoning.

3. B. Kleinmuntz, "The Processing of Clinical Information by Man and Machine," in *Formal Representation of Human Judgment,* ed. B. Kleinmuntz (New York: Wiley, 1968).

4. R. M. Rawes and B. Corrigan, "Linear Models in Decision Making," *Psychological Bulletin* 81 (1974): 95–106.

5. Elstein, Shulman, and Sprafka, *Medical Problem Solving,* 30–36.

6. Two recent and excellent general accounts of the use of computers in medicine are: Benjamin Kleinmuntz, "Medical Information Processing by Computer," in *Computer Diagnosis and Diagnostic Methods,* ed. John Jacquez (Springfield, Ill.: Charles C Thomas, 1972), 45–72; Harold Schoolman and Lionel Bernstein, "Computer Use in Diagnosis, Prognosis, and Therapy," *Science* 200 (1978): 926–931.

7. Schoolman and Bernstein, "Computer Use," 927–928.

8. E. H. Shortliffe, R. Davis, S. Axline, et al., "Computer-based Consultations in Clinical Therapeutics," *Computers and Biomedical Research* 8 (1975): 303–320.

9. H. L. Bleich, "Computer-based Consultation: Electrolyte and Acid-Base Disorders," *American Journal of Medicine* 53 (1972): 285–291.

10. Fred Wiener, "Computer Simulation of the Diagnostic Process in Medicine," *Computers and Biomedical Research* 8 (1975): 132–135.

11. J. Roger Jagoe and Keith A. Paton, "Reading Chest Radiographs for Pneumoconiosis by Computer," *British Journal of Industrial Medicine* 32 (1975): 267–272.

12. T. Allan Pryor, Alan Lindsay, and R. Willard England, "Computer Analysis of Serial Electrocardiograms," *Computers and Biomedical Research* 5 (1972): 709–714.

13. Kleinmuntz, "Medical Information Processing."

14. Malcolm Gleser and Morris Collen, "Toward Automated Medical Decisions," *Computers and Biomedical Research* 5 (1972): 180–189.

15. Goroll, Barnet, Bowie, and Prather, "Teaching Differential Diagnosis by Computer: A Pathophysiological Approach," *Journal of Medical Education* 52 (1977): 153–154. Also Kleinmuntz, "Medical Information Processing," 62–68.

16. Warner, Olmsted, and Rutherford, "HELP—A Program for Medical Decision-Making," *Computers and Biomedical Research* 5 (1972): 65–74.

17. For a system designed to avoid the need of specifying all contingencies in advance (a virtually impossible task, they say) see Pauker, Gorry, Kassirer, and Schwartz, "Towards the Simulation of Clinical Cognition: Taking a Present Illness by Computer," *The American Journal of Medicine* 60 (1976): 981–996.

18. Elstein, Shulman, and Sprafka, *Medical Problem Solving;* also Elstein, Kagan, Shulman, et al., "Methods and Theory in the Study of Medical Inquiry," *Journal of Medical Education* 47 (1972): 85–92. See also Paul Wortman, "Medical Diagnosis: An Information-Processing Approach," *Computers and Biomedical Research* 5 (1972): 315–328 (his emphases are interestingly different from, but compatible with, those of Elstein et al.).

19. Kleinmuntz, "Medical Information Processing," 62.

20. For example, Schwartz, Gorry, Kassirer, and Essig, "Decision Analysis and Clinical Judgement," *The American Journal of Medicine* 55 (1973): 459–472. See also Allen Ginsberg, "The Diagnostic Process Viewed as a Decision Problem," in *Computer Diagnosis and Diagnostic Methods,* ed. Jacquez, 203–240.

21. J. A. Anderson and J. A. Boyle, "Computer Diagnosis: Statistical Aspects," *British Medical Bulletin* 24 (1968): 232–233. They propose a method for dealing systematically with these costs of misdiagnosis. See also Leonard Savage, "Diagnosis and the Bayesian Viewpoint," in *Computer Diagnosis and Diagnostic Methods,* ed. Jacquez, 131–138.

22. A good summary and bibliography of these researchers is Elstein, Shulman, and Sprafka, *Medical Problem Solving,* esp. 30–36.

23. Schoolman and Bernstein, "Computer Use," 927.

24. Anderson and Boyle, "Computer Diagnosis," 234.

25. A. Tversky and D. Kahneman, "Belief in the Law of Small Numbers," *Psychology Bulletin* 76 (1971): 105–110; Tversky and Kahneman, "Availability: Heuristic for Judging Frequency and Probability," *Cognitive Psychology* 5 (1973): 207–232.

26. Schwartz et al., "Decision Analysis," 467.

27. A. Krieg, R. Gambino, and R. Galen, "Why Are Clinical Laboratory Tests Performed? When Are They Valid?" *Journal of the American Medical Association* 233 (1975): 77.

28. See, e.g., Gerald Shea, "An Analysis of the Bayes Procedure for Diagnosing Multi-stage Diseases," *Computers and Biomedical Research* 11 (1978): 65–75.

29. For more on ways of dealing with multiple diseases see John Jacquez, "Algorithmic Diagnosis: A Review with Emphasis on Bayesian Methods," in *Computer Diagnosis and Diagnostic Methods,* ed. Jacquez, 374–393; also

Pauker et al., "Simulation of Clinical Cognition," and Wiener, "Computer Simulation," 129–142.

30. Papers dealing with the dependent symptoms problem: James Croft, "Is Computerized Diagnosis Possible?" *Computers and Biomedical Research* 5 (1972): 351–367; Jacquez, "Algorithmic Diagnosis," 388; Norasis and Jacquez, "Diagnosis I: Symptom Nonindependence in Mathematical Models for Diagnosis," *Computers and Biomedical Research* 8 (1975): 156–172; Norasis and Jacquez, "Diagnosis II: Diagnostic Models Based on Attribute Clusters: A Proposal and Comparisons," ibid., 173–188; Robert Ledley, "Syntax-directed Concept Analysis in the Reasoning Foundations of Medical Diagnosis," in *Computer Diagnosis and Diagnostic Methods,* ed. Jacquez.

31. Marshall B. Jones, "Health Status Indexes: The Trade-off between Quantity and Quality of Life," *Socio-economic Planning Sciences* 11 (1977): 301–305. See also, concerning the assigning of "utility values," David Ransohoff and Alvan Feinstein, "Editorial: Is Decision Analysis Useful in Clinical Medicine?" *The Yale Journal of Biology and Medicine* 49 (1976): 165–168.

32. See K. Danner Clouser and Arthur Zucker, "Medicine as Art: An Initial Exploration," *Texas Reports on Biology and Medicine* 32 (1974): 267–274.

33. Hubert Dreyfus, *What Computers Can't Do: A Critique of Artificial Reason* (New York: Harper and Row, 1978).

2

Typologies of Disease: Nosologies Revisited

H. Tristram Engelhardt, Jr.

In this paper I will explore two general questions: 1) What functions do disease concepts serve? 2) What functions do typologies of disease serve? In addressing these issues, I will narrow my reflections in order to view concepts and typologies of disease with respect to making useful diagnoses. I will argue that for medicine, concepts of disease and typologies of disease are properly therapy-oriented. In contrast, most classifications select one element of what is in fact a network structure of etiological relations and portray that network as a flat hierarchical structure to emphasize one of a set of causal, morphological, or functional considerations.

The history of attempts to provide systematic classifications of diseases is extensive.[1] Though much of the literature has concerned disputes about the characterizations of particular diseases or groups of diseases, there has also been an interest in the more fundamental and philosophical issues of the nature of disease itself. Even this latter enterprise has been undertaken in different fashions. As Kazem Sadegh-zadeh has suggested,[2] the literature concerning the definition of disease reveals at least three general sorts of endeavors: First, there have been attempts to characterize the use of disease language by particular groups of speakers, often physicians or biomedical scientists.[3] For example, one might envisage a linguistic study of the diagnostic language of a particular group—say, of internists or pathologists. A second genre includes more ambitious attempts to seek definitions of disease with reference to essential properties of disease states. Such views hold that definitions of disease are discovered by nonnormative appraisals of physiological functions. This is the position held, for example, by Christopher Boorse,[4] Leon Kass,[5] and von Wright.[6] A third approach is to see the enterprise of defining diseases as one of stipulation. Here the goal is pragmatic. One creates definitions of disease and typologies of diseases partly with a view of their usefulness, that is, by reference to their consequences. This third position is the one that I will defend in this paper. I will put forward an account of diseases, and of typologies of diseases, in which I will sketch some of the purposes built into views of disease and typologies of disease, as well as make some suggestions as to why diseases and nosologies or typologies of disease have been seen in purpose-neutral fashions.

The modern philosophical controversies concerning the standing of disease typologies have turned on the feasibility of defining diseases in terms of physiological functions and dysfunctions. On the one hand there have been well-developed attempts by writers such as Christopher Boorse to show that a nonnormative, neutralist construal of concepts of disease is possible, framed by reference to the species-typical functions of organ systems.[7] These attempts are cast in contrast with normative accounts of disease which presuppose that the proper functions of organs can be specified only with regard to (1) a particular environment and (2) the goals of adaptation within that environment. These normative positions, such as those held by Joseph Margolis and others, do not dispute that there are likely to be great cross-cultural agreements about what should be considered the goals of functioning of certain organs.[8] They have argued, however, that all characterizations of states as being those of health and disease involve evaluations; they involve grading those states—grading them, in fact, with regard to certain chosen standards. Christopher Boorse, on the other hand, has attempted to draw a line between concepts of disease, which he takes to be descriptive and nonnormative, and concepts of illness, which are context- and culture-relative. Thus, he argues that homosexuality is in all circumstances a disease, though it will be an illness in some cultures and not in others, depending on whether it leads to a balance of benefits for the individual involved.[9] He has in mind here a general analysis on the model of an individual declared medically unfit for military service in a war in which the individual does not want to fight. A disease can become a benefit.

If analyses such as those of Boorse succeed, the latitude in creating typologies of disease would be restricted by their having to conform to univocal descriptions of functions and dysfunctions. This, however, involves a second point. In addition to the issue of the normative versus the nonnormative character of disease concepts, there is also the presupposition that disease classifications are natural classifications. If that is not the case, one would be creating typologies on the basis of their usefulness, not strictly in terms of their being the single true typology of diseases or disease phenomena. Typologies could then be distinguished as better or worse by appeal to non-epistemic goals. The issue of the normative versus nonnormative character of disease concepts thus appears on two levels. On the second level, it joins in an ancient dispute in the theory of medicine that has been characterized as a conflict between physiologists and ontologists of disease. With considerable oversimplification of what is at best an incoherent concept, the difference can be put thus: Ontologists of disease held that diseases are enduring clusters of signs and symptoms (though there were also ontologists of disease who simply construed diseases as disease things invading from the outside) and are constellations of pathological findings. It is here that the language of disease entities, *entia morbi,* has its roots. Nosologies would be, then, descriptions of enduring constellations of clinical findings. In contrast, physiologists of disease held that nosologies, and particular disease phenomena, have their boundaries invented, not discovered.[10] All that were real were the laws of physiology. One sorts out some of the expressions of these laws under particular conditions as the clinical presentations of diseases because such sortings and classifications are useful. The ontologists were in that sense realists with regard to their nosologies, while the physiologists were nominalists. The physiologists' view of nosologies, combined with a normative view of diseases, supports the notion that concepts of disease, and the nosologies within which they are placed, are as much invented as discovered.

This view of disease, with some qualifications, is the one that I will adopt for this paper.[11] I hold it because of the impossibility of designating certain physiological phenomena as pathological phenomena without invoking evaluations. An examination of the phenomena brought for medical explanation reveals nondirectly voluntary, physiologically, or psychologically based states judged to be undesirable, in that they (1) are associated with dysteleological conditions—that is, inabilities to perform functions deemed proper to humans of a particular age, circumstances, and sex, (2) are associated with states of pain, or (3) are associated with conditions of deformity or disfigurement.[12] In short, there are a number of medical *explananda* of quite varying character, which we would in ordinary discussions term illnesses, sicknesses, diseases, deformities, injuries, dysfunctions, defects, or medical complaints. These conditions that bring individuals to physicians I will stipulatively term states of illness, in order to contrast them with various explanatory accounts proffered by physicians and others to account for these explananda. Such states of "illness" can include angina, pain at childbirth, fever, pain while teething, anxiety—in short, first- or third-party complaints that bring individuals to medical care. The explanations of these phenomena may be etiological, functional, structural, or some similar sort of attempt to explain why the identified typologies of complaints occur as they do, and why and how they should be treated. In short, there are, in contrast with descriptive typologies of complaints, various *explanatory typologies of complaints*. These explanatory typologies, following a suggestion from nineteenth-century approaches, can be stipulatively referred to as *diseases*, though this genus will include explanations of processes underlying complaints which we would not in ordinary language refer to as diseases (e.g., the physiological and anatomical basis of pain at childbirth).

These views have implications for the meaning and structure of typologies of disease. Devising typologies of illness and disease becomes an open-ended endeavor if the goal is to generate a classification of what brings people to physicians or causes others to bring people to physicians so that their complaints can be better treated in virtue of the typology. This is the case in part, for what counts as a complaint turns on culturally dependent value judgments. In addition, there is more than one defensible way of viewing typologies of disease insofar as their organizations are directed toward different therapeutic goals. One might think here of how one could try to specify exactly at what point a subclinical encounter with mycobacterium tuberculosis should be counted as an illness, as well as whether tuberculosis should be construed as a genetic, social, or infectious disease. The first would be an issue of defining illnesses, the second of classifying diseases.

This two-tiered world of illness and diseases, of phenomena to be explained and explanations of medical phenomena, became full-blown in the nineteenth century through the work of such men as Xavier Bichat (1771–1802),[13] François-Joseph-Victor Broussais (1772–1838),[14] Rudolf Virchow (1821–1902),[15] and Carl Wunderlich (1815–1877).[16] It became possible to relate the world of the clinician to a second world, that of the pathophysiologist and pathoanatomist. As I will suggest, one constructs the relations to the second world in terms of which typologies of explanation turn out to be more or less useful.

One should note also that the generation of this two-tiered world of the clinician and the pathophysiologist led to a view in the nineteenth century that the second tier captures the true essence of disease. This occurred in part because more accurate pathophysiological and etiological accounts of disease allowed one to reorganize usefully the world of clinicians. Thus, for example, typhoid could be resolved into two clinical "entities," one caused by a bacterium, typhoid, and another by a rickettsia, typhus.[17] Other clinical complaints that had not been associated could be brought together under one rubric. For example, phthisis and scrofula could both be recognized as manifestations of tuberculosis. This led as well to the notion that treating the underlying pathophysiological disorders should be counted as real medicine, for it involved etiological treatment, while merely treating the symptoms (i.e., symptomatic treatment) was less scientific.

Much of this development has been sketched in engaging and helpful detail by Michel Foucault in his book, *The Birth of the Clinic.*[18] It should be noticed, however, that the movement from the clinically oriented medicine of the eighteenth century to the pathoanatomical medicine of the twentieth century hardly counts as the birth of the clinic. This development led (1) to discounting the importance of clinical accounts, (2) to viewing the underlying pathoanatomical changes as the real diseases, and (3) to suggesting the feasibility of simply discovering, rather than also in part inventing, the typologies of disease.

To summarize to this point, I have stressed the heterogeneity and complexities of views of disease and of the classification of diseases. For example, typologies of medical problems tend to mix typologies of complaints with typologies of explanations of complaints. In the terms I have suggested, they mix typologies of illness with typologies of disease. Moreover, both are structured in a weak-normative fashion. Classifications of illnesses turn on various gradings, evaluations of objective events in the world; classifications of diseases turn in part on the usefulness of different ways of explaining and acting upon complaints. An appreciation of how the worlds of complaints and of diseases are played off against each other in nosologies can be gleaned from comparing the complaint-oriented nosologies of eighteenth-century medicine with our more etiologically and pathoanatomically oriented typologies of medicine.

In the eighteenth century, under the influence of Thomas Sydenham's (1624–1689) concept of natural histories of diseases,[19] numerous clinicians attempted to classify complaints in order to give a basis for prognosis and treatment undistorted by various physiological theories of disease. That is, these clinicians classified patient complaints as they appeared to the clinician for the purpose of maximizing effective care. The result was an attempted phenomenology of the world of the physician. This approach had many presuppositions, including the rationality of appearance (i.e., that phenomena present themselves in univocal constellations of signs and symptoms which can be systematically studied). As a result, there were numerous clinical typologies of diseases (for these classifications the boundary between illnesses and diseases is difficult to discern). An excellent example is the 1763 nosology of Carolus Linnaeus (1707–1778), his *Genera Morborum* (1763).[20] Linnaeus placed diseases under eleven classes: (1) rashes, (2) phenomena characterized by crises, (3) inflammations, (4) pains, (5) disturbances of mentation, (6) decreases in activity, (7) motor disturbances, (8) suppressed activities, (9) evacuations, (10) deformities, and (11) defects.

A classical nosology in the genre was also provided by François Boissier de Sauvages de la Croix (1707–1776) in his *Nosologia Methodica Sistens Morborum Classes, Genera, et Species, juxta Sydenhami Mentem et Botanicorum Ordinem* (1768).[21] As the title suggests, Sauvages attempted to erect a typology of diseases on the basis of Sydenham's presupposition that clinical findings fell into easily identifiable clusters that can be recognized through their natural histories. Moreover, he held that one can classify diseases as one can plants, by reference to similarities and dissimilarities in morphology and development. The result was a taxonomy of some 2400 species of clinical findings arrayed within 315 genera, placed under 42 orders, and finally displayed within 10 classes of disease. Since Sauvages explicitly wished to eschew as far as possible reference to causal, including physiological, accounts in framing a nosology, what one finds is a geography of the world of the clinician. That is, his typology of diseases was erected in order to allow unambiguous diagnoses by clinicians and to assist them in making reliable prognoses and in engaging in successful therapeutic endeavors. In contrast with Foucault's account of this matter, the endeavor was far from being a wooden rationalism. Sauvages recognized that the characterization of the species of disease should be based on experience with patients and, somewhat pragmatically, that the genera should be given a stable meaning even if such clarity is not fully found in the data. Such coherence would be sought in order to guide treatment, as is suggested by Cullen's *Nosologia,* which functioned as a guide to therapy.[22]

However, the world of Sauvages's clinicians stands in stark contrast with our world, which is structured at least in part by reference to the world of the pathoanatomist. Sauvages's classes of disease were, for example, (1) impairments, (2) fevers, (3) inflammations, (4) spasms, (5) difficulties in breathing, (6) debilities, (7) pains, (8) madnesses, (9) fluxes, and (10) wastings. Thus, hemorrhages, abortions, leukorrhea, and gonorrhea all fell under the class of "fluxes." What were important were the major clinical signs presented to the physician—something was flowing. This attitude remained even in the very influential classification of William Cullen (1710–1790) in *Synopsis Nosologiae Methodicae* (1769).[23] He, for example, placed diseases in a typology that allowed for four classes: (1) febrile states, (2) neuroses, (3) wastings, and (4) local disturbances.[24] Since his was primarily a clinical typology of disease, it had room for such disease entities as simple and complex nostalgia.[25] States of affairs were clinical problems if they were not directly under the control of the patient, were in principle amenable to medical manipulations, and were implicitly due to some physiological or psychological disturbance. However, no particular lesion was required in order to authenticate a complaint. Thus, Sauvages had a category of disease *dolores vagi qui nomen a sede fixa non habent.*[26] As a result, the worried well properly fell under the aegis of medicine and were not to be viewed, as our post-nineteenth-century prejudices incline us to view them, as crocks, as individuals without a canonical complaint.

An inspection of current classifications of disease shows in contrast a heavy admixture of concepts from pathology, microbiology, and physiology. For example, the *Systematized Nomenclature of Pathology,* put forward by the College of American Pathologists, offers four different modes of classifying diseases: (1) topographical classification, (2) morphological classification, (3) etiological classification, and (4) functional classification.[27] These rubrics are intended to facilitate the uniform recording of areas of information concerning diseases. In fact, the *Systematized Nomenclature* views these four rubrics as four distinct, though interdependent, modes in terms of which diseases may be defined. It is important here as always to remember the envisaged function of the typology—in this case, to aid pathologists in maintaining records in which there is a standardization of terms and therefore an increased efficiency in the classification and storage data concerning diseases. The typology thus is seen as a propaedeutic to the acquisition of better pathoanatomical information concerning diseases and disease processes.

One finds a similar heterogeneity in the *International Classification of Diseases,*[28] which is aimed as well at the acquisition of better information concerning the incidence, prevalence, and character of diseases. Again a standardized language for diagnosis is sought. As one would suspect, the rubrics of the typology are heterogeneous and include such classes as infective and parasitic diseases; neoplasms; endocrine, nutritional, and metabolic diseases; diseases of the blood and blood-forming organs; mental disorders; diseases of the nervous system and sense organs; diseases of the circulatory system; diseases of the respiratory system; diseases of the digestive system; diseases of the genitourinary system; complications of pregnancy, childbirth, and the puerperium; diseases of the skin and subcutaneous tissue; diseases of the musculoskeletal system of connective tissue; certain causes of perinatal morbidity and mortality; symptoms and ill-defined conditions (including such conditions as nervousness and debility); accidents, poisonings, and violence—internal causes; accidents, poisonings, and violence—external causes (including such conditions as legal executions and injury due to war operations involving nuclear weapons). The foregoing classification thus mixes together etiological, morphological, functional, and topological considerations. Such a heterogenous array of categories, however, is by no means misguided, for it is serving the important purpose of standardization of medical data, a goal sought as well by the nosologists of the eighteenth century. In fact, if one looks at these volumes, and others such as the American Medical Association's *Current Medical Information and Terminology,*[29] one sees an ongoing attempt to standardize medical diagnoses and information gathering, which is expressed as well in such regimens as Laurence Weed's Problem-Oriented Medical Record.[30] These differ (Weed's proposal excepted) from many of the eighteenth-century nosologies, in that they are not immediately tied to a clinical problem.

It is this difference between eighteenth- and twentieth-century typologies which is most striking in that one of the possible services of a typology of disease is assistance in medical decision-making, not only in developing reliable diagnoses but in effecting useful treatment of clinical problems. Modern typologies are, however, not usually seen to have this close relationship to clinical interests except for the *Diagnostic and Statistical Manual* of the American Psychiatric Association, which is bereft in many sections of the usual etiological and other independent reference points by which to clarify syndromes.[31] Still, some of the more encompassing proposals concerning the classification of diseases have in mind questions of alternative classifications for possible alternative therapies. One might think here of proposals in the psychiatric literature concerning the advisability of somatic, psychological, behavioral, and sociological modes of approach to diseases.[32] One should, though, note that these proposals often conflate the issue of different models of therapy with the issue of different ways of classifying diseases. What is at stake, frequently, is a somewhat different dispute, one concerning whether one should have a medical or nonmedical approach to the care of individuals— whether, for example, one should place particular groups of individuals within a sick role. But arguments concerning the classification of diseases as somatically or physically caused are of interest here in that these discussions indirectly signal the important service that typologies can offer. Classifications can indicate which therapeutic approach is likely to be the most successful or on balance the most cost-effective in time, money, and patient vexation. Consider, for example, whether one lists tuberculosis as an infectious disease, a genetic disease, an environmental disease, or one of defective immunity. We signal tuberculosis as an infectious disease in that this appears to indicate the most efficient mode of treating and preventing the condition. There is evidence, however, that there are genetic variations in the susceptibility of populations to tuberculosis.[33] We know little of the precise genetics of differences in resistance or susceptibility to tuberculosis, and in any case a eugenics program aimed at increasing resistance to tuberculosis would very likely be more dangerous than would be justified. Similar considerations influence the categorization of tuberculosis as an immunological failure or as a disease due to social conditions. With regard to the latter, for instance, there is a great deal of information that general social variables bearing on housing and nutrition affect the morbidity and mortality patterns of tuberculosis.[34] The point is that nosologies of disease can signal where or how one should think about treatment or prevention. *Sub specie aeternitatis,* however, any classification of any particular disease is liable to have an arbitrary character, not unlike Sauvages's collecting of hemorrhages and gonorrhea under the class of fluxes.

This point can be appreciated by an inspection of the numerous, well-accepted medical conditions of unknown or complex etiology. In many of these conditions classifications of the disease states are made with relative disregard of their etiological basis in favor of a classification that signals the most appropriate immediate therapeutic approach. Consider, for example, appendicitis. The diagnosis identifies the culmination of various and obscure causal processes, which processes can be effectively ignored in favor of a classification that indicates where in general the surgeon should incise and remove inflamed tissue. It is a pathoanatomical classification. An etiological classification would be beside the point. The same is true of a great number of other diagnostic categories in surgery, and it holds for conditions addressed by other specialties as well.

Etiological classifications are likely to be embraced, however, if they can be tied to therapy, especially since they possess an allure given the hope for specific therapies for specific diseases. Consider, for example, what is likely to happen to the classification of neoplasms if it were to be established that in one class of neoplasms there is an important causal role played by viruses and a virally oriented treatment for such malignancies becomes available. And imagine as well that there is another class of neoplasms that comes to be recognized as for the most part causally dependent upon the effects of particular chemical carcinogenic agents and for which a treatment becomes available that can prevent or even reverse the effects of such substances. Neoplasms would, given such circumstances, be classified in one case as infectious diseases and in the other case as diseases due to chemical agents. This is likely to hold even if a strong genetic component were to be established in both instances.

The point is that effective typologies of disease do serve, and should serve, not only the interests of coherent data collection but those of therapeutic decision making as well. There has, however, been very little thought about how typologies of disease can be aimed at therapeutic goals and how such typologies would need to be structured. Any attempt to realize these goals would probably lead to a very complex classification, designed on the one hand to display likely problems of differential diagnosis and on the other hand to signal likely therapeutic options. Such a classification would probably not be subject to display in tabular form, but would exist as a nexus comprehended in a program for clinical decision making.

Endeavors of this sort exist at present only in fragments. One might think here of the progression in a clinician's use of disease classification from diagnosing a patient as having a fever to asserting that the patient has rheumatic fever (obvious ambiguities should at once leap to mind, for this could involve as well an increase in determination regarding the classification of arthritis or choreiform movements). The classic criteria for the diagnosis of rheumatic fever, as proposed by T. Duckett Jones, offered two alternate means of establishing grounds for asserting that an individual has rheumatic fever.[35] It was suggested that one should hold that a diagnosis had been established once either two major manifestations of the disease or one major and two minor manifestations had been demonstrated. Major manifestations were taken to include carditis, polyarthritis, chorea, erythema marginatum, and subcutaneous nodules. Minor manifestations included a previous history of rheumatic fever or rheumatic heart disease, arthralgia, fever, increased erythrocyte sedimentation rate, the presence of C-reactive protein, leukocytosis, and a prolonged P-R interval in the electrocardiogram. If one questions why it is reasonable to require only two major and not three, or why some other relation of major and minor manifestations would not be better, the answer must be in terms of what are taken to be the costs of false positive and false negative diagnoses. As the treatment becomes more effective and has fewer sequelae, and the disease becomes more serious, one is likely to make the diagnosis easier and require fewer indications, or have less stringent conditions that must be met to make the diagnosis. That is, one has fewer grounds to avoid false positive diagnoses and stronger reasons to wish to prevent false negative diagnoses. One would be more concerned about individuals undiagnosed who would not receive helpful treatment (i.e., imagining that effective treatment existed for rheumatic fever). One could thus imagine a typology in which the fanning out of the branches of its tree of classifications represented further credible moves to greater clinical intervention, and where the threshold for the movement to a more precise classification is set to reflect an appreciation of the various costs of treating and not treating. However, because of the complexity of the etiological, pathoanatomical, pathophysiological, and pathopsychological considerations that would be required, one would have a nexus much more involved than the *Systemized Nomenclature of Pathology* which the College of American Pathologists has proposed for the domains of topographical, morphological, etiological, and functional data.[36]

What I have been suggesting here is a proposal for constructing various alternate typologies of disease, aimed at facilitating different sorts of clinical decision-making. On this point I agree in great measure with Henrik Wulff's suggestion that disease categories be regarded as vehicles of clinical knowledge and experience, shaped toward the goal of better treatment.[37] It is in this sense that typologies of disease are not *true or false* in any straightforward fashion but rather are more or less *useful* in the conduct of clinical medicine. The lines of classification are, in short, as much invented as discovered, where the criteria for good inventions must in the end be based upon the typologies in the treatment and prevention of disease. Along this line one must attend to criticisms such as Alvan Feinstein's of the *Standard Nomenclature of Diseases and Operations*[38] and of the *International Classification of Diseases*.[39] He asserts that such classifications may press a clinician to be more specific in his or her description of a patient's state than the data justify. Feinstein, for example, defends the clinical category of *stroke* against the more precise terms *cerebral arteriosclerosis* or *encephalopathy*.[40] One might think here as well of the recognized fragmentation by the *Systematized Nomenclature of Pathology* of clinical entities such as Wilson's disease into such terms as *copper disorder, ceruloplasmin disorder*, and *hepatolenticular degeneration*.[41] The point again is that a typology of disease must be clinically employable and therapeutically useful.

This leads to the following general conclusion: One should develop classifications of disease with a view to maximizing the achievement of the goals of treatment and prevention. Since most disease states are multiply caused and can be viewed in varying ways with regard to cause, morphological changes, and disturbances of function, one should choose among these possibilities on the basis of the alternative costs and benefits of different classifications. This view of disease and typologies of disease is consistent with the complaint-oriented nature of the institution of medicine. It should be clear that since such typologies are structured to achieve certain goods and avoid certain harms (e.g., to effect an "acceptable" balance of goods and harms from certain rates of false positives and false negatives), they are far from simply descriptive or explanatory. They involve unannounced value judgments regarding what constitutes prudent balances of possible benefits versus possible harms. A typology of diseases can systematize such judgments. The enterprise of developing nosologies can thus be understood as directed toward the better achievement of the goals we have in mind from medicine. One should describe the clinical world in anticipation of the consequences of some descriptions versus the consequences of other descriptions (i.e., diagnoses) for the good of the patients one is likely to treat. Evaluations of anticipated consequences of explanations will thus influence the explanations and descriptions, the diagnoses one proffers. In the development of diagnoses and general orderings of diagnoses (i.e., typologies of disease, nosologies), evaluations and explanations are intimately intertwined.

NOTES

1. Knud Faber, *Nosography in Modern Internal Medicine* (New York: Hoever, 1923).

2. Kazem Sadegh-zadeh, "Krankheitsbegriffe und nosologische Systeme," *Metamed* 1 (1977): 2.

3. Horacio Fabrega, Jr., "Disease Viewed as a Symbolic Category," in *Mental Health: Philosophical Perspectives,* ed. H. T. Engelhardt, Jr. and S. F. Spicker (Dordrecht: Reidel, 1976), 79–106.

4. Christopher Boorse, "Health as a Theoretical Concept," *Philosophy of Science* 44 (December 1977): 542–573.

5. Leon Kass, "Regarding the End of Medicine and the Pursuit of Health," *The Public Interest* 40 (Summer 1975): 11–24.

6. Georg Henrik von Wright, *The Varieties of Goodness* (New York: Humanities Press, 1963).

7. Christopher Boorse, "On the Distinction between Disease and Illness," *Philosophy and Public Affairs* 5 (Fall 1975): 49–68.

8. Joseph Margolis, "The Concept of Disease," *The Journal of Medicine and Philosophy* 1 (1976): 238–255; also H. T. Engelhardt, Jr., "Ideology and Etiology," ibid., 256–268. A comprehensive discussion of these issues is provided in *Health, Disease, and Causal Explanations in Medicine,* ed. Lennart Nordenfelt and B. J. B. Lindahl (Dordrecht: D. Reidel, 1984).

9. Boorse, "Disease and Illness," 63. See also Christopher Boorse, "Health as a Theoretical Concept," *Philosophy of Science* 44 (1977), 542–573. One should note that Boorse has modified his views. He now holds that

even concepts of illness are value-free. See Boorse, "On the Distinction between Disease and Illness," in *Concepts of Health and Disease,* ed. A. L. Caplan, H. T. Engelhardt, Jr., and J. J. McCartney (Reading, Mass.: Addison-Wesley, 1981), 560.

10. Here *ontologist* and *physiologist* are used in a special sense to indicate adherence to what have been termed ontological or physiological views of disease. See, e.g., Owsei Temkin, "The Scientific Approach to Disease: Specific Entity and Individual Sickness," in *Scientific Change,* ed. A. C. Crombie (London: Heinemann, 1961), 629–647; also Henry Cohen, *Concepts of Medicine,* ed. Brandon Lush (Oxford: Pergamon Press, 1960); Peter H. Niebyl, "Sennert, van Helmont, and Medical Ontology," *Bulletin of the History of Medicine* 45 (March–April 1971): 115–137.

11. H. Tristram Engelhardt, Jr., "The Concepts of Health and Disease," in *Evaluation and Explanation in the Biomedical Sciences,* ed. H. T. Engelhardt, Jr. and S. F. Spicker (Dordrecht: Reidel, 1975), 125–141.

12. H. Tristram Engelhardt, Jr., "Human Well-Being and Medicine: Some Basic Value-Judgments in the Biomedical Sciences," in *Science, Ethics, and Medicine,* ed. H. T. Engelhardt, Jr. and D. Callahan (Hastings-on-Hudson: Hastings Center, 1976), 120–139.

13. Xavier Bichat, *Anatomie général appliquée à la physiologie et la médicine,* 4 vols. (Paris: Brosson, Gabon, 1801).

14. François-Joseph-Victor Broussais, *Examen des doctrines médicales et des systèmes de nosologie,* vol. 2 (Paris: Méquignon-Marvis, 1824).

15. Rudolf Virchow, *Disease, Life, and Men,* trans. Leland Rather (Stanford: Stanford Univ. Press, 1958).

16. Carl Wunderlich, "Einleitung," *Archiv für physiologische Heilkunde* 1 (1842): i–xxix.

17. One of the last important treatises identifying typhus and typhoid as one disease was written by William Stokes, *Lectures on Fever* (London: Longmans, Green, 1874).

18. Michel Foucault, *The Birth of the Clinic: An Archaeology of Medical Perception,* trans. A. M. Sheridan Smith (New York: Random House, 1973).

19. Thomas Sydenham, *Observationes Medicae circa Morborum Acutorum Historiam et Curationem* (London: Kettilby, 1676).

20. Carolus Linnaeus (Carl von Linné), *Genera Morborum* (Uppsala, Sweden: Steinert, 1763).

21. François Boissier de Sauvages de la Croix, *Nosologia Methodica Sistens Morborum Classes, Genera, et Species, juxta Sydenhami Mentem et Botanicorum Ordinem* (Amsterdam: de Tournes, 1768).

22. Ibid., vol. 1, #100, p. 18; William Cullen, *Nosologia Methodica* (Edinburgh: Carfrae, 1820).

23. William Cullen, *Synopsis Nosologiae Methodicae* (Edinburgh: Creech, 1769).

24. Cullen, *Nosologia Methodica* (see above, n. 22).

25. Ibid., 152.

26. Sauvages de la Croix, *Nosologia Methodica*, vol. 1, 94.

27. Committee on Nomenclature and Classification of Disease, *Systematized Nomenclature of Pathology* (Chicago: College of American Pathologists, 1969).

28. World Health Organization, *Manual of the International Statistical Classification of Diseases, Injuries, and Causes of Death, Based on the Recommendations of the Eighth Revision Conference, 1965, and Adopted by the Nineteenth World Health Assembly* (Geneva, 1967–1969); U.S. National Center for Health Statistics, *International Classification of Diseases, Adapted for Use in the United States*, 8th revision, Public Health Service Publication no. 1693 (Washington, D.C.: U.S. Government Printing Office, 1967–1969).

29. American Medical Association, *Current Medical Information and Terminology* (Chicago: American Medical Association, 1971).

30. Lawrence Weed, *Medical Records, Medical Education, and Patient Care* (Cleveland: Case Western Reserve Press, 1969).

31. American Psychiatric Association, *Diagnostic and Statistical Manual of Mental Disorders*, 2d ed. (Washington, D. C.: American Psychiatric Association, 1968) (DSM-II).

32. Aaron Lazare, "Hidden Conceptual Models in Clinical Psychiatry," *The New England Journal of Medicine* 288 (1973): 345–351.

33. M. B. Lurie, "On the Mechanism of Genetic Resistance to Tuberculosis and Its Mode of Inheritance," *Human Genetics* 4 (1953): 302–314; K. Planansky and G. Allen, "Heredity in Relation to Variable Resistance to Pulmonary Tuberculosis," *American Journal of Human Genetics* 5 (1953): 322–349.

34. René Dubos, *Man Adapting* (New Haven: Yale University Press, 1965).

35. T. Duckett Jones, "The Diagnoses of Rheumatic Fever," *The Journal of the American Medical Association* 126 (1944): 481–484; Committee on Standards and Criteria for Programs of Care of the Council of Rheumatic Fever of the American Heart Association, "Jones Criteria (Modified) for Guidance in the Diagnosis of Rheumatic Fever," *Modern Concepts of Cardiovascular Disease* 24 (1955): 291–293; Ad Hoc Committee to Revise the Jones Criteria (Modified) of the Council on Rheumatic Fever and Congenital Heart Disease of the American Heart Association, "Committee Report: Jones Criteria (Revised) for Guidance in the Diagnosis of Rheumatic Fever," *Circulation* 32 (1965): 664–668.

36. See above, n. 27.

37. Henrik R. Wulff, *Rational Diagnosis and Treatment* (Oxford: Blackwell Scientific Publications, 1976).

38. American Medical Association, *Standard Nomenclature of Diseases and Operations* (New York: McGraw-Hill, 1961).

39. See above, n. 28.

40. Alvan R. Feinstein, *Clinical Judgment* (Huntington, N.Y.: Krieger, 1974), 968.

41. *Systematized Nomenclature of Pathology* (see above, n. 27), xvii.

3

Artificial-Intelligence Approaches to Problem Solving and Clinical Diagnosis*

Herbert A. Simon

I was asked to speak about the relation of artificial intelligence to medical diagnosis. As my paper developed, however, I realized that I was poaching on the territory of the session scheduled to precede this one, for my remarks are mainly about the nature and philosophy of medical diagnosis itself. Since I was presumably invited to this conference for my expertness on AI, and certainly not for my expertness on medical matters, which is nonexistent, I feel I have to offer at least a brief explanation of why my analysis took the course that it did.

Artificial intelligence is not very different from the real thing. (In fact, in my book *The sciences of the artificial* [1981] I argued that all intelligence belongs to the realm of the artificial.) Intelligence, whether natural or artificial, is directed toward the use of symbols, and of information processes applied to symbols, in order to solve problems. The methods available for doing this often depend much more on the nature of the problem-solving task and its environment than upon the characteristics of the problem solver—provided that the problem solver

*This research was supported by Research Grant MH-07722 from the National Institute of Mental Health.

is a more or less serial information-processing system, as both computers and people are.[1] To be sure, computers can store and retrieve numbers faster than people can, and perform much more elaborate arithmetic operations on them, but the asymmetry in the other direction is not nearly as striking. Increasingly, computers can be programmed to do the things that people do, using much the same methods that people use.

So with artificial intelligence (and now I mean machine intelligence) we have a choice. We can use the computer's speed, arithmetic capabilities, and vast memories to solve problems in ways that people cannot, or we can construct programs that imitate, more or less closely, the problem-solving methods we find people using.

Elements of both of these approaches are represented in the automated medical-diagnosis schemes I shall discuss. People probably do not use anything closely resembling Bayesian decision theory in making diagnoses. They probably do use processes that are somewhat more akin to the twenty-questions schemes and the causal-linkage schemes that I will develop below. I do not want to imply, by the way, that we have good empirical evidence as to exactly how people make diagnoses. The assertions I have just made are based on what we know in general about human information-processing capabilities and what we have learned about human problem-solving methods by studying chess playing, puzzle solving, theorem proving, and similar performances.[2]

But the same issues must be faced in evaluating a diagnostic procedure, independently of whether it is humanoid or not. Does it call for unconscionable amounts of computation? Does it rest on a sound view of the diagnostic task? Is it highly reliable? The contents of a paper on "Artificial-Intelligence Approaches to Diagnosis" would not need to be much changed if the first two words of its title were eliminated.

The one difference that is consequential relates to the phrase *unconscionable amounts of computation*. As I have already remarked, computers are able to carry out computations that would be utterly impossible for people. Hence, the range of design alternatives for an artificial-intelligence system to do diagnosis is wider than the range for people. From the very beginnings of artificial-intelligence research, the relative extents to which one should rely on machine power versus the imitation of human cunning has been a central issue.

The initial impulse has usually been to exploit the computer's great comparative advantage in speed of symbol manipulation and to build brute-force schemes that would solve problems by undertaking vast amounts of search. Such schemes have often been swallowed up by the exponential expansion of the problem space with deeper and deeper search. This occurred, for example, in the 1960s in the case of chess-playing programs and programs for proving mathematical theorems.

The exponential explosion of the search space is countered by intro-ducing selectivity—in either or both of two ways. On the one hand (as occurred in the case of theorem proving) the task domain may have a deep mathematical structure and correspondingly strong formal prop-erties. These formal properties may be exploited by introducing rules for searching only part of the space without danger of missing the solution. A good example is the use of the simplex method to solve linear programming problems, which exploits certain properties of convexity and linearity to search only a small set of the boundary points of the space of feasible solutions.

The other route to selectivity is to give up absolute guarantees of reaching the exact solution and to resort to various rules of thumb, or heuristics, as they are now usually called, that direct search to the most promising regions of the search space. A good example is the use of expert chess knowledge to incorporate a plausible move generator in a chess program, so that not all moves will have to be examined but only those that give promise of being good moves.

The history of artificial intelligence in realms like theorem proving and chess (chess has been the *Drosophila,* the standard laboratory organism of the field) has been a continuing dialectic between machine power, on the one hand, and these two means for achieving selectivity, on the other. Moreover, there has been no clear verdict for the supe-riority of either approach. As the potentiality of machine speed is exhausted, design moves toward new forms of selectivity. As machine technology moves forward rapidly to new levels of speed and memory capacity, the balance moves backward again. The best contemporary chess-playing programs (which have now reached the level of master play) find both speed of computation and chess knowledge indispens-able. They look at enormous numbers of different possibilities (hun-dreds of thousands or even millions), which are, however, only a tiny fraction of the legally admissible continuations of the game. The history of theorem-proving efforts has gone through the same oscilla-tions and taught the same lessons.

With these introductory comments out of the way, let me now turn to the specific topic of medical diagnosis. Space does not permit me to review the whole range of medical-diagnosis programs that have been proposed, or actually constructed, in the past twenty years. Instead I will organize my discussion in terms of the main conceptual frameworks that have been used in the design of such systems: problem solving, tree search, statistical decision theory, causal analysis, and biological modeling. The reader who wishes to learn more about early efforts in medical diagnosis by computer will find excellent surveys in Ledley 1962 and Kleinmuntz 1969. As for recent work, Szolovits and Pauker (1978) have provided a thoughtful comparison of four of the most prominent current systems: PIP, INTERNIST, CASNET, and MYCIN. Most of the literature of the field is listed in the bibliographies of one or another of these three sources.

DIAGNOSIS AS PROBLEM SOLVING

In one of their papers on the INTERNIST system for medical diagnosis (then called DIALOG), Pople, Myers, and Miller (1975) questioned whether diagnosis is problem solving at all. Instead, they suggested, it should be regarded as "problem formulation" or "problem finding." I am going to disregard their suggestion and try to characterize medical diagnosis as a form of problem solving, as that term is used in the discipline of artificial intelligence. I think this is a disagreement only in terminology and not in substance, but if I am mistaken in that, Harry Pople can correct me when it comes his time to speak.

The usual definition of a problem runs like this (Newell and Simon 1972, 74): Given a set U, to find a member of a subset of U having specified properties (called the goal set, G). As a first approximation in the case of medical diagnosis, we can take U as the set of all possible disease entities, G as the disease present in a particular patient (or the collection of his diseases, if he has more than one), and the "specified properties" as the indications, for example, a pathologist would use on autopsy to determine what the disease "really was." The performance of an autopsy is not the critical element here but the presence of some retrospective, hindsight evidence that enables the correct diagnosis to be pinned down. Perhaps G is most simply conceived in terms of an omniscient being who holds not only a full knowledge of the patient's condition but a complete and correct theory of human physiology as well. In practice we have to settle for the autopsy as an approximation to this omniscient being.

Now the information that is available to identify members of G is a set of manifestations or symptoms, ascertainable by examining the patient and/or submitting him to laboratory tests. A *complete* examination would disclose for the patient the presence or absence of every possible manifestation. The possibility of medical diagnosis rests on the premise that there is a unique mapping (a function) from sets of manifestations to disease entities. Notice that a particular disease entity, in this formulation, may manifest itself in different ways, but a particular (complete) set of manifestations can point to only a single disease, or to a set of discriminable diseases from which the patient is suffering simultaneously.

There is nothing simple about the mapping of symptoms on diseases. There are two main complications. First, a patient may be suffering from several diseases, all of which are to be identified from the symptoms. Second, individual symptoms may be unreliably associated with a disease, so that an accurate diagnosis can be made only on the basis of a constellation of manifestations, any single element of which may be present or absent in a particular instance of the disease. This second complication is often described as "unreliability" or "noisiness" of the symptomatic information, but I have treated it here as a matter of incompleteness rather than inaccuracy. (Nature cannot be inaccurate in describing herself, but she can be coy.)

Of course, this rather formal characterization of diagnosis conceals the medical import of what is going on in the process. The physician is not interested in arbitrary mappings from sets of manifestations to labels called "disease entities." The latter have the further significance for him that they map onto alternative courses of treatment. The latter mapping may be pragmatic—it is known that a certain disease entity can usually be treated successfully with certain medication—or it may be based on a more or less deep understanding of the etiology of the symptoms. In either event the symptom-disease mapping is not arbitrary but reflects knowledge of treatment possibilities and/or the etiology of diseases. I will have a good deal to say about these points a little later.

DIAGNOSIS AS TWENTY QUESTIONS
OR STATISTICAL DECISION THEORY

The view of diagnosis as mapping symptoms onto diseases conceptualizes it as a taxonomic process, which might be organized and carried out as other taxonomic tasks are, in biology and elsewhere. Note that it is not the task of the diagnosis to *discover* the taxonomy of disease; that is presumed to be already given. Discovering and classifying disease entities and their identifying manifestations is quite a different task—an interesting and important one, but not one with which we will be concerned here.

If we are given a taxonomy and asked to apply it to specimens, how do we go about it? A time-honored method (you can find it exemplified, for example, in your Gray's *Botany*) is the "twenty-questions" strategy: construct a taxonomic key that prompts the user down a branching list of questions the answers to which discriminate successively among groups of species until a unique identification has been made.

(For examples of applications of the twenty-questions approach to medical diagnosis, see Kleinmuntz 1969, 244–260.)

The twenty-questions strategy provides a not implausible basis for designing a medical-diagnosis program. Such a program would be large but not enormous. I suppose that there are not more than tens of thousands of identified distinct disease entities (fewer, say, than the number of distinct species of beetles in the United States). The number of dichotomous questions that would have to be asked, if the asking were organized efficiently, to identify a specimen in a system of N species is only $\log_2 N$, where $\log_2$ is the logarithm to base 2; and the total number of questions in the twenty-questions tree is only N.

Moreover, there are various possibilities for organizing the tree efficiently. Questions that are cheaply and safely answered (e.g., that don't require expensive or dangerous laboratory tests) can be asked first, and the questioning stopped as soon as a unique diagnosis has been made.

Why, then, have we not long since constructed a twenty-questions scheme to automate once and for all the process of medical diagnosis? We shall see presently that there are a number of reasons why this might not work very well, and why we probably would not be satisfied with it even if it did. But we shall see also that there is a good deal of the twenty-questions philosophy embedded in the existing successful medical-diagnosis schemes. In fact, the improvement of these schemes over earlier versions may lie less in their departures from the twenty-questions strategy than in the fact that they embody larger data bases of manifestations and diseases and more accurate and sophisticated mappings of the former onto the latter than did their predecessors.

The main reason usually given for departing from the simplest twenty-questions strategy is that symptoms are unreliable and noisy.

A symptom, S, of disease D may be present in only some fraction of cases of D, and may also be present in some (usually smaller) fraction of cases of diseases other than D. This quite correct observation leads almost inexorably to the idea that the linkages between symptoms and disease entities should be expressed as probabilities. And it is only one step from viewing these linkages as probabilistic to the idea that the whole task of diagnosis should be represented as a problem in statistical decision theory instead of a twenty-questions problem.

Decision-theoretic strategies are based upon Bayes' theorem.[3] Every disease entity is conceived to have a certain probability of occurrence. When a patient appears in the physician's office, and before he has been examined, he is assumed to have disease D_i with probability P_i. This probability is the so-called *prior* probability of Bayesian theory. (The "evoking-strength" parameter in INTERNIST plays roughly the role of a prior probability in that system.) There is nothing very questionable about such an assumption: actuarial tables of all sorts represent calculations of probabilities of exactly this kind. Moreover, in a well-designed Bayesian system it will turn out that the final diagnoses are quite insensitive to the exact values that are assigned to these prior probabilities. Mainly, they just provide a way to get the decision system started, so to speak.

At the next step we must assign to each symptom-disease pair, S_i, D_j, a conditional probability that if a patient is suffering from disease D_j, he will exhibit symptom S_i. We can represent this conditional probability as $P(S_i/D_j)$. (In INTERNIST the "import" parameter plays the role of this conditional probability.) Now if we know the values of these probabilities for all symptom-disease pairs, and if we know for a given patient which symptoms he is exhibiting (and which he is *not* exhibiting), we can calculate the posterior (conditional) probability, $P(B_j/S_1, \ldots S_N)$, that he is suffering from disease B_j. The calculation is based straightforwardly on Bayes' formula, which I have no need to reproduce here (see Szolovits and Pauker 1978, 119). We can then identify the patient's condition with the disease entity that has the highest posterior probability.

A number of questions about the practicality and even the validity of this scheme come readily to mind. First, in building the data base, all the symptom-disease probabilities must be estimated. If there are, say, 10^4 different disease entities and 10^4 manifestations (I don't know whether these numbers are realistic, but they are probably in the ballpark), then there are 10^8 probabilities to be estimated. Perhaps, however, all but a few of them are very small and can be set equal to zero. Second, in applying the scheme to the individual case the presence or absence of each symptom must be determined (at least in principle) and the values of all the nonvanishing probabilities for the pairs inserted in the formulas. Observe that the formula for the calculation includes the probability of the *absence* of each symptom, when it is found to be absent, as well as the probability of its presence, when present. Clearly the Bayesian formula involves a great deal more computation than going down a simple decision tree.

But I don't want to exaggerate the practical difficulties. Numbers like 10^8 strike no terror into the heart of a modern computer. The best existing chess-playing programs, of master caliber, often examine several million possibilities before choosing a move, and do it in a matter of ten minutes or so. Many of us would regard a medical decision as comparable in importance with the choice of a chess move, and would not begrudge fifty dollars of computer time if that would guarantee its accuracy. Moreover, the symptom-disease linkages can be computed once and for all; they do not have to be recalculated for each individual case but can be simply plugged into Bayes' formula to compute the posterior probability for that case for each disease. This is a more modest task than estimating the linkages themselves.

However, there are problems with the Bayesian analysis that go beyond computational difficulties. In the form in which it is usually used in diagnosis, the Bayesian formula assumes that the various conditional probabilities, $P(S_i, D_j)$, appearing in numerator and denominator are independent—that the presence or absence of one symptom does not affect the probability of the presence or absence of another. As has often been noticed, this is an unlikely assumption. In fact, we might well expect to find situations where the presence of a particular symptom is indicative of a disease in the presence of a second symptom but counterindicative in the absence of the latter.

To handle the problem of nonindependence of the conditional probabilities in its most general form, we should have to estimate not merely the probability of linkage between each symptom-disease pair but the probability of linkage between each possible *set* of symptoms and each disease. With N symptoms and M diseases, that would require the estimation of 2^NxM probabilities, a formidable number even for N of modest size. As a practical matter, of course, we would not expect very many of the interactions to be important, but that is an empirical question to be decided on the basis of the evidence and not a priori.

Thus the proper mode of application of Bayes' theorem to medical diagnosis is far from obvious, and in point of fact, it has seldom been incorporated in its pure, unadulterated form in medical-diagnosis programs. Rather, it has been used as a conceptual guide to the general shape of the program. In many if not most such programs there appear weights associated with symptoms that can be given at least metaphorical interpretation as Bayesian conditional probabilities. These "probabilities"—perhaps it would be better to call them "plausibilities" or "confidence indicators"—are then manipulated to produce judgments of the plausibility that the patient is suffering from one or another disease. The final diagnosis corresponds to the disease with highest a posteriori plausibility.

Having reached this point, we can show that any result reached by a Bayesian scheme, even a sophisticated one taking account of the nonindependence of the conditional probabilities, can be reached in a quite straightforward way with a twenty-questions scheme. Although we introduced the probabilities to take care of the unreliability of individual symptoms, the twenty-questions game can also be played in such a way as to handle noisy data. Let us see how this can be done.

The result of a Bayesian analysis is to rank disease entities according to their posterior probabilities in the light of the manifestations that are present and absent. The diagnosis assigns to the patient the disease or diseases highest on the list. For any given configuration of symptoms (i.e., presence or absence of all possible manifestations) the system will always assign the same probabilities and reach the same diagnosis. At the last step in the process the uncertainty disappears from it and the system makes some yes-or-no judgments.

Now we could construct a simple table, with no probabilities whatsoever, associating with each symptom configuration the appropriate diagnosis (i.e., the diagnosis that would be assigned by the Bayesian procedure). We could also construct a decision tree for searching that table and could endeavor to "optimize" the decision tree so that diagnoses could be reached after the smallest possible numbers of tests. The decision tree arrived at in this way would normally be larger than the one we would construct if our data were noise-free. We would be using the redundancy deriving from the large number of alternative manifestations of disease to eliminate the unreliability of depending upon individual symptoms.

I must emphasize that the diagnoses obtained with this decision-tree method would be identical with those reached by the Bayesian method. (We could even use the Bayesian method as the first step in the construction of the decision tree.) The actual diagnostic process, however, would involve the computation of no probabilities or numerical weights, but a simple twenty-questions procedure.

Now if we questioned a diagnostician who was using a decision tree, we might discover that he was, after all, a crypto-Bayesian. At a certain branching in the tree he might argue that certain disease entities could be ruled out as "extremely improbable in the light of the configuration of symptoms." If he felt uncertain about a diagnosis because of the unreliability of symptoms, he could always exploit the redundancy of nature by adding a few "confirming tests" to his diagnostic tree. It is a nice philosophical question, which we probably don't have to answer here, whether the decision tree is simply a crystallized form of a Bayesian analysis or whether a Bayesian analysis is simply a rationalization of a decision tree. I myself lean toward the latter alternative. In self-observation I seldom catch myself calculating numerical probabilities, conditional or otherwise, and my observations of my fellow men do not suggest that they (or I) are capable of much arithmetic.

Before I leave the topic of statistical diagnosis, one other theoretical issue should be discussed. We have framed the decision problem (and so have the Bayesian diagnostic systems with which I am familiar) as if the task were to maximize the probability of reaching the correct diagnosis. Of course that is not what medicine is about at all. The diagnosis is simply a step toward treatment, and we would be perfectly willing to be wrong about the diagnosis as long as we were right about the treatment. More specifically, there are consequences attached to taking the right or the wrong measures (and not simply to making the right or the wrong diagnoses), and some of these consequences are far more serious than others.

In statisticians' language, there are errors of two kinds: errors of accepting a hypothesis when it is false and errors of rejecting it when it is true. Suppose that a diagnostician is faced with the choice between disease A, which can be treated safely and effectively but which is fatal unless treated, and disease B, for which there is no good treatment but which also has no serious consequences. The choice between diagnosing a mole as malignant (A) or nonmalignant (B) would be a case of this kind. With equal probabilities on the evidence for both diagnoses, or even with a somewhat higher probability that B was the correct diagnosis, the diagnostician would be advised by decision theory to choose A—that is, to act as if the patient were suffering from A. Without the advice of statistical decision theory, the intelligent diagnostician would probably have arrived at the same conclusion. He has almost nothing to lose, even if he chooses A erroneously, and almost everything to gain if he avoids choosing B erroneously.

To convert the usual Bayesian scheme into a statistical decision scheme taking account of consequences, we simply have to attach to each diagnosis numerical values representing the respective costs of the two kinds of errors. Then, instead of selecting the diagnosis that has the highest probability, we select the one that minimizes the expected loss from a mistake. The same kind of consideration of risks can be introduced into a decision-tree procedure, again without making the risks explicit, or representing them numerically.

DIAGNOSIS AS CAUSAL ANALYSIS

The approaches to diagnosis that have been discussed in the previous section represent a purely Baconian point of view. They incorporate no real theory of disease, only a set of empirical correlations between congeries of manifestations and disease entities. And a disease entity is itself a purely pragmatic construct: all the combinations of symptoms that yield to the same course of treatment may just as well be mapped onto a single disease entity. A disease, in such a scheme, has no existence apart from its symptoms and its treatments.

This Baconian representation is probably not an entirely unsatisfactory description of the approach of traditional medicine, which operated with nearly a complete lack of knowledge of physiological mechanisms, if with a somewhat better knowledge of anatomy. There are probably substantial areas of contemporary medicine where it is only a moderate caricature of the conceptualizations that are used, particularly if we look at everyday clinical practice rather than medical research.

But Baconian systems don't satisfy us very deeply, whether in artificial intelligence, medical diagnosis, or science in general. We wish to know not only *that* certain things happen but *why* and *how* they happen. We would like to have a reasoned account of the relation between symptoms and disease. Lacking such understanding, we will hardly regard a taxonomic scheme as exhibiting intelligence, no matter what its practical utility may be. Thus, in modern taxonomic systems in biology, we are not satisfied to put species close together simply because they resemble each other in some arbitrary ways. Instead we seek a classification that reflects phylogeny, commonality of origins. We want not just any old tree but the actual family tree.

The impulse toward explanation is not solely aesthetic. When strong theories are discovered, theoretical explanations are usually far more parsimonious, more powerful in prediction, and often more accurate than empirical correlations. Hence, we prefer the former to the latter when we can discover them. Of course it is a question of fact, in any particular domain and at any given stage of development of that domain, whether the available theory is actually more useful than the known empirical regularities. I shall return to this issue, as it applies to various domains of artificial intelligence, in a later section.

Let us see how we might introduce more theory—more intelligence—into a system for medical diagnosis. The first step amounts to a change in terminology. Instead of conceiving symptoms as being associated with disease entities, we think of them as being *caused* by diseases. That does not change our symptom-disease linkages, but it does induce us to interpret them a little differently and in the opposite direction from the previous one. Further, it takes one step toward realism, for it allows us to conceive of diseases as causing not only symptoms but other diseases as well. Hence, we can incorporate disease-disease links into the scheme, as has been done, for example in INTERNIST. Now, in cases where a patient is diagnosed as having more than one disease, we need not regard these as independent (although they may be) but can look for causal links between them. This will be important in treatment, where we will generally want to work upstream from symptoms to their fundamental causes.

The causal links can, like the correlation links they replace, be empirically determined, or they can reflect such theoretical understanding as we have of mechanisms. Although I don't know that this has been done, it would be perfectly possible to associate with each link in the system a theoretical account of the reason for that link—which might include an account of reasons for its unreliability. This might be an especially valuable feature in a system for teaching diagnosis if not in a clinical diagnostic system.

Interpretation of the symptom-disease links as causal suggests a different diagnostic procedure from the Baconian one we have described thus far. Instead of homing in on a diagnosis by step-by-step elimination of possibilities or by making a comparative Bayesian evaluation of alternative possibilities, we can proceed in two steps, usually referred to as *hypothesis* and *test*. In the first step, prominent symptoms are used to evoke or hypothesize one or more candidate disease entities. In the second step, the hypotheses are tested by following the causal linkages in the reverse direction, testing whether the symptoms are present that would be expected to be present if the candidate disease were the actual cause of the pathology. INTERNIST makes important use of the hypothesis-and-test method (Pople, Myers, and Miller 1975).

Similar procedures, based on causal analysis, have cropped up in other domains of artificial intelligence, and have been observed, also, in human problem-solving behavior in complex task environments. A major finding of de Groot's (1946, 1978) pioneering studies of chess grand masters was that the grand master, facing the task of selecting a move, rather quickly but tentatively chose a "favorite," then spent most of the rest of his time verifying that the favorite was indeed a good move. Sometimes, of course, a flaw revealed itself in the course of the evaluation, and then another favorite had to be selected. In the very first seconds of his examining a new position, the grand master identified the three or four plausible candidate moves from which he then chose the favorite. This initial identification of plausible moves was made, it would appear, on the basis of prominent "diagnostic" features of the position that could be detected by a skilled player in a few seconds' examination of the board.

The process described by de Groot differs only a little from the simplest hypothesize-and-test process. The hypothesizing is preceded by a very rapid *recognition* process, which may be regarded as a preliminary hypothesis-identification step based on the most obvious symptoms present. If these symptoms fail to point to the correct hypothesis among those selected for examination, then the validation step must be sufficiently thorough to detect the error and enlarge the set of candidate hypotheses.

Causal Linkages versus Biological Models

The network of nodes representing disease entities and symptoms, with the links between them interpreted causally, may be viewed as a primitive model of the etiology of disease. The model does not represent the normal working of the system but only deviations from normality. A disease refers to some subsystem that is behaving pathologically, and symptoms are the consequent pathological values of observable variables. Moreover, the model is very weak. It postulates connections between certain variables, but it does not have much to say about the strengths of those connections—the coefficients that we are accustomed to see modeled in a dynamic system. The model is also abstract. It does not represent organ systems (e.g., the heart or the lungs) directly, nor the main physiological processes (e.g., respiration, digestion). Of course, particular symptoms and particular diseases may be totally or largely confined to particular organs or processes, but this is implicit in the model. There is no explicit anatomy or physiology in it.

Hence, while the causal model is, I think, a genuine biological theory, it does not much resemble the formal mathematical models that we are accustomed to build of systems—and which generally do provide an explicit representation of their concrete structure or at least their organization in terms of processes.[4] On the other hand, this causal theory may be very much like the qualitative commonsense theories that we use in everyday life to reason about the complex systems with which we have to deal. Unless we are automobile mechanics, I would venture that our model of the operation of our car is of just this abstract kind. That is just a hunch; I know of no empirical evidence on this point, and it would be very useful to gather some.

Let me provide a contrasting example of a different kind of model used in an artificial-intelligence system that was designed to handle diagnostic processes. John Seely Brown and his associates constructed a program, SOPHIE, to teach troubleshooting analysis of electronic circuits (Bobrow and Brown 1975). One component of SOPHIE is a set of equations for an actual, rather complex, circuit. Various malfunctions (diseases) can be introduced into the circuit by changing certain parameters (e.g., short circuits) or by rendering certain components inoperative. These malfunctions can be detected by reading the values of certain other circuit variables (symptoms). The student's task is to diagnose the malfunction by examining the symptoms and by making tests (altering various control variables) that could disclose other symptoms. SOPHIE is sufficiently sophisticated to be aware of the structure of the circuit, and can not only report to the student the results of the tests he performed but also tutor him by offering advice as to new observations and tests he could make.

The SOPHIE model, in contrast with the causal-link models, contains a full quantitative theory of the normally operating system. Malfunctions and symptoms are represented as deviations from these normal values. The model is so constructed that the malfunctions do in fact induce, or cause, the symptoms: it actually behaves in a causal manner exactly as the real circuit would behave. Moreover, the various components of the modeled circuit can be identified as corresponding components of the mathematical model. Instead of using a system of inference rules to explore the consequences of the causal connections, SOPHIE simply solves and re-solves the equations of the system as the independent variables are manipulated. Straightforward numerical calculations replace qualitative inference rules as the tool of causal analysis.

The contrast between a node-link causal structure and a SOPHIE-like system, between reasoning inferentially about causality and modeling the causal structure of a system, has long been of interest in artificial intelligence (Pople 1972; Simon 1972). The usual laws of the predicate calculus do not apply to reasoning about sentences containing causal language. McCarthy and Hayes (1968), among others, have attempted to construct special modal logics to handle causal predicates, but without great success. Simon (1972) has shown that the difficulties encountered are not superficial but are bound to arise whenever there are complex interactions among the components of the system under discussion (e.g., the nonindependence of the Bayesian probabilities). In the presence of such interactions a modal logic will be either too weak (will fail to support some valid inferences) or too strong (will permit invalid inferences). Nothing short of full modeling, in the manner of SOPHIE, will handle correctly all of the interactions of a complex system; and the tool of inference used with such a model is ordinary mathematical reasoning, that is, higher-order predicate calculus (Simon 1977).

The fact that only approximate relations in complex systems can be represented by causal-link models is not a condemnation of such models, which may, as experience with medical-diagnosis systems has shown, have great heuristic value. In fact, Pople (1972) has constructed a GOL system that is capable both of modal reasoning and of model simulation. Its inferential machinery can be used to suggest hypotheses that are then tested by manipulation of the model.

If validity of inferences cannot be guaranteed in a causal-link scheme, one might suppose that such schemes would be dubious mechanisms for medical diagnosis, where reliability is a main desideratum. When such a system is used in hypothesize-and-test mode, however, the unreliability of inferences can be overcome by providing redundancy in symptoms. Stated otherwise, the causal linkage is not relied upon completely to reach definitive diagnosis but principally as a means of discovering candidate hypotheses for further consideration. By subsequently accumulating evidence until one hypothesis is favored decisively, protection is obtained against relying too heavily on single chains of inference.

I do not wish to imply that the theoretical issues surrounding causal inference are all thoroughly understood. On the contrary, this is an area in which further clarification would be both welcome and important for the future development of the theory and practice of diagnosis and taxonomy.

Earlier I mentioned the utility of causal linkages for following symptoms "upstream" to their instigating conditions. From the standpoint of scientific curiosity and understanding we of course want to get as close as we can to fundamental causes. From the therapeutic or "troubleshooting" standpoint we want to follow the causal stream up to a point where intervention is possible. In the face of certain symptoms we might conclude "cirrhosis of the liver" or "alcoholism." Which is the more useful diagnosis will depend upon the means at our disposal for correcting the patient's bodily functions or changing his habits.

Similar issues of localization of cause—to identify the precise spot for intervention—have arisen in a variety of artificial-intelligence systems. Pfefferkorn (1975), for example, constructed a system for arranging furniture or equipment in a room, subject to various relational constraints. The several items were sited one by one. If an impasse was reached, so that no appropriate location could be found for the next item, a causal analysis was instituted to find which items were causing the trouble (i.e., which constraints were hard to satisfy). The search was then reinitiated, reordering the items so as to site the difficult ones first.

Designers of chess-playing programs are increasingly turning to causal analysis to avoid unnecessary analysis of worthless moves (Berliner 1977). When a sequence of moves under investigation leads to a poor result, the sequence is not simply abandoned. Instead a causal analysis is initiated to trace the disaster upstream in order to identify the specific move in the sequence that was responsible for the poor outcome. If this move can be identified, then the other possible sequences of play descending from it need not be investigated but can be discarded without search.

Finally, there is a close connection between causal reasoning and the means-ends analysis that is the backbone of many artificial-intelligence problem-solving schemes. The idea of means-ends analysis is that if there is a set of differences between the current situation and the goal situation, appropriate operators should be applied to remove these differences, one by one (Newell and Simon 1972). The operator is the means for removing the difference (which is the end). The relation between operator and difference is clearly causal. Hence, means-ends search can be interpreted as heuristic causal inference. It does not escape the usual inadequacies of modal causal inference—that is, the inability to handle interactions—for it assumes that the differences can be removed independently, one at a time. Combined with best-first search methods, however, it has proved to be a powerful heuristic tool in a variety of problem-solving environments.

THE EVALUATION OF
DIAGNOSTIC SYSTEMS

As in other domains of artificial intelligence, the initial goal of research on automated medical diagnosis has been to demonstrate feasibility, by constructing systems actually capable of making diagnoses at an acceptable quality level. The task has been to prove an existence theorem, so to speak. Since I think it fair to say that this has now been accomplished, several new tasks lie ahead. An obvious one is to improve the systems we have and bring them into actual application, in some symbiotic relation with the human components of the medical system, to improve medical technology.

Another task, complementary to the first, is to understand why these systems work and to see what light they may cast, both on the nature of the diagnostic process and on the theory of artificial intelligence. Work toward those goals has hardly begun. Let me remind you of some of the main issues, which have already emerged in the course of my discussion.

The Knowledge Base

The best existing diagnostic schemes now provide us with an answer to the question of how much medical knowledge needs to be incorporated to yield diagnoses of professional quality. The answer (similar to the one we are getting in other applications of AI to professional problems) is "a great deal, but not an unmanageable amount." That is a rather vague answer: what it means is that the knowledge required is well within the memory capacities of modern computers and that the number of man-years of effort required to transfer the knowledge to those memories is quite moderate, even with our present crude methods for doing so.

We do not know how much the performance of a program like INTERNIST would be improved if it had an order-of-magnitude more knowledge at its disposal, nor, I suspect, do we quite know how it could use that additional knowledge at all.

Choice of Methods

Up to the present time, little *systematic* effort has been devoted to exploring the relative efficacy of different basic methods. That is not to say that a wide variety of AI methods has not been employed in different medical-diagnosis schemes. Many of them, in fact, have been quite eclectic, with features borrowed from the twenty-questions, statistical-decision-theory, and causal-linkage schemes. So far as I am aware, no existing system uses biological modeling techniques more complex than causal linkages.

What has not been investigated systematically, and what we do not know, is the relative contribution of these several components to the effectiveness of the systems. Among other difficulties in making such comparisons, no two systems have even remotely comparable data bases. In fact, a real case could be made for the position that it is the steady elaboration of the data bases, rather than the sophistication of the problem-solving methods, that has accounted for most of the progress in automatic medical diagnosis. The data bases, even the most complete, are hardly large enough to strain the capabilities of modern computers using relatively unsophisticated and unselective search methods. This is, of course, only a hypothesis, since we simply do not have the experimental data about comparative system performance that would permit us to test decisively whether it is correct.

The size of the search space in medical diagnosis does appear, however, to be considerably smaller than the spaces in either chess or speech recognition. In both of those domains, sophisticated search has had to be combined with computing power to reach the goal. Moreover, in chess there has been enough experience with a variety of systems (Berliner 1977), and in speech recognition enough systematic exploration of a family of systems (HEARSAY and HARPY among others: see Walker et al. 1977), to give us a pretty good feel for the improvement in performance that would be bought with either an increment of machine speed or an increment of selectivity.

My remarks about the dearth of performance data on medical-diagnosis systems should not be interpreted as criticism of the research that has been going on in this field. I would suppose that the total effort to date can be measured in terms of dozens, rather than hundreds or thousands, of man-years' work. That is a far cry from a moon shot or a Manhattan Project, and there is no more reason to expect costless miracles in this research domain than in any other.

Medical Diagnosis and Biological Theory

It is always something of a disappointment in AI research when brute-force schemes or simple-minded selective procedures do the job. The disappointment is quite irrational, of course, but it does have several understandable roots. First, we would prefer the challenge of conceptualizing sophisticated techniques and capturing them in our programs. Second, we are always reluctant to concede that high-level human professional performances, that are achieved only after years of training and experience, can be imitated or replaced by simple programs.

Pride in human accomplishment should not blind us to the facts, however. A growing body of experience in AI, over a considerable number of task domains, points increasingly to the possibility that it is the size and quality of his data base more than the sophistication of his methods for analyzing evidence that distinguishes the expert from the novice. This does not mean that the methods themselves or the organization of the data base are unimportant. It may mean that a small repertory of general methods, several of which have been discussed in this paper, are adequate to handle a wide range of professional data bases.

If this is true, or even partly true, it has implications for the relation of fundamental biological theory to clinical practice. Even if we could model the human anatomy and physiology in some detail, and run our models dynamically, it is not clear that we would want to use such models directly for diagnostic purposes. They would be too detailed, too elaborate, too cumbersome for that. What is more likely is that we would extract from the models their important qualitative properties and convert these into systems of causal linkages that we could incorporate into our diagnostic-reasoning schemes. In its "ultimate" form the automatic diagnostic system would not be organized very differently from the causal-link schemes we are beginning to have today.

This may be a general paradigm for the relation between theory and practice and for the way in which theory gets incorporated into everyday professional analysis and reasoning. Of course there are exceptions. In civil engineering, at least in the final stages of design, we do employ the laws of mechanics directly, model our systems mathematically, and solve the equations explicitly. But the limited number of domains that are simple enough, and well enough understood, to permit us to do this may not provide the correct paradigm for the uses of theory in other parts of science. In any event the domain of medical diagnosis appears to be a promising field in which to explore the alternative design that I have sketched above.

NOTES

1. Of course both the eye and the ear are parallel information-processing systems, but there is little evidence for parallel processing in the central nervous system, once the initial perceptual encoding of sensory stimuli has been accomplished. Since diagnosis systems are not concerned with that initial encoding, we may treat such systems as essentially serial in their operation. For further discussion see Simon 1979.

2. See Newell and Simon 1972; Simon 1979.

3. Good brief explanations of Bayesian statistical analysis applied to medical diagnosis can be found in Ledley 1962, 342–344, and in Szolovits and Pauker 1978, 119–122.

4. For an example of explicit modeling of the circulatory system, see Guyton et al. 1973.

REFERENCES

Berliner, H. 1977. Search and knowledge. In *Proceedings of the Fifth International Joint Conference on Artificial Intelligence*, 975–979. Pittsburgh: Dept. of Computer Science, Carnegie-Mellon University.

Bobrow, R. J., and J. S. Brown. 1975. Systematic understanding: Synthesis, analysis and contingent knowledge in specialized understanding systems. In *Representation and understanding*, ed. D. Bobrow and A. Collins. New York: Academic Press.

de Groot, A. D. 1946. *Het denken van den schaker*. Amsterdam: North-Holland.

————. 1978. *Thought and choice in chess*. 2d. ed. The Hague: Mouton. Revised translation of de Groot 1946.

Guyton, A. C., T. G. Coleman, A. W. Cowley, K. W. Scheel, R. D. Manning, and R. A. Norman. 1973. Arterial pressure regulation. In *Hypertension manual*, ed. J. H. Laragh. New York: Dun-Donnelley.

Kleinmuntz, B. 1969. *Clinical information processing by computer*. New York: Holt, Rinehart & Winston.

Ledley, R. S. 1962. *Programming and utilizing digital computers*. New York: McGraw-Hill.

McCarthy, J., and P. J. Hayes. 1968. Some philosophical problems from the standpoint of machine intelligence. In *Machine intelligence 4*, ed. B. Meltzer and D. Michie. Edinburgh: Edinburgh University Press.

Newell, A., and H. A. Simon. 1972. *Human problem solving*. Englewood Cliffs, N.J.: Prentice-Hall.

Pfefferkorn, C. 1975. The design problem solver. In *Spatial synthesis in computer-aided building design*, ed. C. M. Eastman. London: Applied Science Publishers.

Pople, H. E. 1972. A goal-oriented language for the computer. In *Representation and meaning*, ed. H. A. Simon and L. Siklossy. Englewood Cliffs, N.J.: Prentice-Hall.

Pople, H. E., J. D. Myers, and R. A. Miller. 1975. DIALOG: A model of diagnostic logic for internal medicine. In *Proceedings of the Fourth International Conference on Artificial Intelligence*. Cambridge, Mass.: Artificial Intelligence Laboratory, M.I.T.

Simon, H. A. 1981. *The sciences of the artificial*. Cambridge, Mass.: M.I.T. Press.

————. 1972. On reasoning about actions. In *Representation and meaning,* ed. H. A. Simon and L. Siklossy. Englewood Cliffs, N.J.: Prentice-Hall.

————. 1977. *Models of discovery,* chap. 3.1. Dordrecht: Reidel.

————. 1979. *Models of thought.* New Haven: Yale University Press.

Szolovits, P., and S. G. Pauker. 1978. Categorical and probabilistic reasoning in medical diagnosis. *Artificial Intelligence* 11:115–144.

Walker, D. E., L. D. Erman, A. Newell, N. J. Nilsson, W. H. Paxton, T. Winograd, and W. A. Woods. 1977. Speech understanding and AI. In *Proceedings of the Fifth International Joint Conference on Artificial Intelligence.* Pittsburgh: Department of Computer Science, Carnegie-Mellon University.

4

Steps toward Mechanizing Discovery

Bruce G. Buchanan

INTRODUCTION

This is the thirtieth anniversary of the publication of Professor Hempel's landmark in the philosophy of science, "Studies in the Logic of Explanation." Because this paper is about computer programs that generate explanations, my debt to Professor Hempel will be obvious.[1] However, insofar as I wish to use the term *discovery* to cover the activity of finding explanations, I know that Professor Hempel will not entirely agree with these ideas about mechanizing the activity.

The purpose of this paper is to elaborate a very simple idea: that discovery in science and medicine can be profitably viewed as systematic exclusion of hypotheses. That is, hypotheses that explain empirical data can be found systematically by methods that can be implemented in computer programs. The conditions under which this view makes sense are an important part of the elaboration. Two necessary conditions are that the space of relevant hypotheses is definable and that there exist criteria of rejection and acceptability. Because the space of hypotheses is immense for most interesting problems, it is also desirable that there exist criteria for guiding a systematic search. This idea was voiced recently by Linus Pauling, in an interview about his creative work:

> So what I'm saying is, it's important to have a big background of knowledge. Also to do a lot of thinking. Probably part of the secret of being successful in a field involving discovery is the sort of judgment that keeps you from working in the wrong direction. A student once asked me, "Dr. Pauling, how do you go about having good ideas?" and I answered, "You have a lot of ideas and you throw away the bad ones."
> [13]

Kenneth Schaffner has argued [18] that scientific discovery and justification have essentially the same logic, in the sense that the forms of inference and the scientific norms are the same in both cases. His carefully reasoned study of a major discovery in molecular biology leads him to the conclusion that "essentially the same forms of inference and general types of considerations or factors can be used in searching for a new hypothesis, i.e., in generating it, as can be used to assess and criticize or defend it after the hypothesis is found." Consistently with Schaffner's conclusion, this paper argues that many of the *same* criteria used to judge a hypothesis can be used as constraints on the hypothesis generator. Moreover, the decision to use information during generation rather than testing is based on extralogical considerations such as cost, convenience, and efficiency. The feasibility of implementing these ideas in a computer program is demonstrated in the second half of this paper by describing existing programs that formulate hypotheses in organic chemistry and molecular genetics.

Computer Programs as Models

We turn to computer programs as illustrations because their methods are necessarily explicit (although not always clear). We are not proposing that the traditional dream of an *infallible* method for investigating nature scientifically will be realized through computer programming. It is unlikely that a machine will ever be programmed to do induction in the same straightforward way and with the same guarantees that it can be programmed to add a column of figures, for instance. A program can, however, reason symbolically using inexact methods in problem areas for which infallible methods are missing. There are numerous examples in which numerical algorithms fail to provide satisfactory explanations in science and medicine. For solutions to these kinds of problems, we turn to a branch of computer science known as heuristic programming.

Heuristic programs differ from other computer programs in the extent of the guarantees they impart to their conclusions. A heuristic program, as distinguished from an algorithm, has been characterized as "a process which may solve a given problem, but offers no guarantees of doing so" [15]. Polya describes heuristics in a similar way: "Heuristic reasoning is reasoning not regarded as final and strict, but as provisional and plausible only, whose purpose is to discover the solution to the present problem" [16].

HEURISTIC SEARCH AS A METHOD OF DISCOVERY

Searching for a Hypothesis

In general, the problem for a discovery method is twofold: (1) to choose a language, L, in which to express hypotheses, explaining data in a scientific domain, and (2) to choose a satisfactory sentence of L that explains the data. In paradigm revision, to use Kuhn's terms, the first half of the problem is crucial, for the choice of the language establishes boundaries on the factual content of the paradigm. Choosing to speak of light as traveling (Toulmin's example [22]) determines in large measure the kinds of questions we ask about light and the kinds of answers the paradigm will furnish.

On the other hand, choosing a language is not part of the problem of finding an explanation in normal science or clinical medicine, for the language in which hypotheses are expressed is just the language of the current paradigm. That is, once a paradigm is established, scientists routinely describe their work within that language; only when description and explanation within the language of normal science fail does a scientist again face the problem of choosing a new language in which to express hypotheses. At this point we will not discuss the problems of choosing a language, although I will return to it at the end.

The second half of the problem—choosing one of the sentences in

L to serve as a hypothesis—is a problem that a logic of discovery might help solve. The problem addressed here is to find efficient methods for picking out sentences of L that are most likely to succeed as hypotheses in a given case. A grossly inefficient method is to generate the sentences of L, say in lexicographic order, and test each one. It is clear that scientists do not resort to an enumeration and one-by-one trial of sentences of L, for we would expect no progress in science with such inefficiency. For similar reasons, exhaustive enumeration of hypotheses by a computer is out of the question for all but trivial problems.

As an alternative we could consider discovery to be merely successful guessing, as is often suggested, and program a machine to generate hypotheses randomly—perhaps restrained within the correct subject area. It could test each random hypothesis against the criteria of success and stop when a hypothesis met those criteria. Although some inquiring minds may work in this random manner, it hardly recommends itself as a rational method. In addition, neither random search nor exhaustive enumeration carries any sense of terminating when there is *no* sentence in L that meets the criteria.

Heuristic Search

The method of systematic exploration sketched above is very like the old method of induction by elimination. Solutions to problems can be found and proved correct, in this view, by enumerating possible solutions and refuting all but one. Obviously the method is used frequently in contemporary science and medicine, and is as powerful as the generator of possibilities. According to Laudan, however, the method of proof by eliminative induction, advanced by Bacon and Hooke, was dropped after Condillac, Newton, and LeSage argued successfully that it is impossible to enumerate exhaustively all the hypotheses that could conceivably explain a set of events [12]. The force of the refutation lies in the open-endedness of the language of science. Within a fixed language the method reduces to *modus tollens.*

The computational method known as heuristic search is in some sense a revival of those old ideas of induction by elimination, but with machine methods of generation and search substituted for exhaustive enumeration. Instead of enumerating all sentences in the language of science and trying each one in turn, a computer program can use heuristics enabling it to discard large classes of hypotheses and search only a small number of remaining possibilities. Heuristic search is the best-known and most widely used method underneath symbolic reasoning programs. It has been applied, with some variations, in problem areas ranging from chess to chemistry and from mathematics to molecular genetics. The method depends essentially on heuristics, or rules of thumb, that guide the search for hypotheses and set the criteria for plausibility of hypotheses.

The key ideas behind heuristic search are:[2]

a) implicitly define the complete space of hypotheses within language L;
b) define a stepwise generator of progressively more precise hypotheses within this space;
c) during generation, eliminate incorrect or implausible classes of hypotheses;
d) after generation, test the generated candidates in order to eliminate some and rank the rest.

There are many ill-defined terms in this characterization. Instead of discussing alternative definitions, however, I will illustrate the use of heuristic search in three computer programs that formulate explanatory hypotheses in science.

Heuristic DENDRAL

Two sets of computer programs developed at Stanford University use heuristic search for hypothesis formation in organic chemistry and thus constitute an empirical demonstration of the feasibility of the ideas advanced here. These programs are called Heuristic DENDRAL and Meta-DENDRAL. They are closely related but work at two different levels of scientific activity. Another program that reasons about molecular genetics will be discussed later.

Both programs are organized around the heuristic-search method in which relevant hypothesis spaces are searched systematically under heuristic constraints. The fundamental assumption is that discovery can be viewed as systematic exclusion of hypotheses from a mechanical hypothesis generator. In all interesting problems the hypothesis space is so large that the *heuristics* must be powerful enough to exclude large classes of hypotheses before they are generated and the *generator* must be flexible enough to exclude classes of hypotheses under many different descriptions.

This methodology requires (1) a constructive definition of possible hypotheses that can be used as a generator of items in the hypothesis space (steps a and b above) and (2) criteria for selecting and rejecting classes of hypotheses (steps c and d above). The discussions of the two programs focus on these two requirements.

All of these programs are predicated on the assumption that finding scientific hypotheses can be treated in much the same way as other cognitive problems and does not require unique solution methods. Problem solving in science, including hypothesis formation, has many of the same information processing characteristics as problem solving in other areas [17].

The Heuristic DENDRAL program [3][3] is designed to aid organic chemists in determining the molecular structure of organic compounds from empirical data. The observed data for an unknown compound are *explained* in the sense that once the correct molecular structure is hypothesized, the data can be predicted from the deductive application of a theory (of the analysis technique) to the hypothesized chemical structure.

Inferring structural information from empirical data generally requires a thorough understanding of the instrument or technique that produced the data.[4] For example, the reasons for noisy, ambiguous, or missing data, as well as the origins of data points, must be factored into the interpretation. The value of an analytical procedure in chemistry lies in its ability to provide information about the composition and structure of the unknown compound. For example, a chemist wants to know about the presence or absence of oxygen in the unknown, the number of oxygen atoms doubly bonded to carbon atoms, the sizes of rings, and so on, in order to determine the topological structure of the molecule.

Structure Elucidation with Constraints from Mass Spectrometry

Parts of the Heuristic DENDRAL program have been highly tuned to work with experimental data from an analytical instrument known as a mass spectrometer. (See [6] for technical details.) Mass spectrometry is a new and still developing analytic technique. It is not ordinarily the only analytic technique used by chemists, but is one of a broad array, including nuclear magnetic resonance (NMR), infrared (IR), ultraviolet (UV), and "wet chemistry" analysis. It is particularly useful when the quantity of the sample to be identified is very small, for mass spectrometry requires only micrograms of sample.

A mass spectrometer bombards the chemical sample with electrons, causing fragmentations and rearrangements of the molecules. Charged fragments are collected by mass. The data from the instrument, recorded in a histogram known as a mass spectrum, show the masses of charged fragments plotted against the relative abundance of the fragments at each mass. Although the mass spectrum for each molecule may be nearly unique, it is still difficult to infer the molecular structure from the 100–300 data points in the mass spectrum because, not only does a spectrum contain "noise peaks" and overlapping peaks originating from many parts of the molecule, but the theory of mass spectrometry is not complete.

Determination of molecular structure is mostly a task within routine science, in Kuhn's term again; no new terms or relations need to be postulated to account for the data. Occasionally new techniques are invented that allow identification of more classes of compounds. But these new techniques are quite readily assimilated by the routine scientists making the identifications.

Generating Hypotheses

The DENDRAL generator of molecular structures (named CONGEN for Constrained Generator) is the heart of the whole program. The problem description it starts with is a list of chemical atoms (including the number of atoms of each type) together with constraints on the ways groups of atoms can and cannot be associated. The language in which hypotheses are expressed, and generated, is the so-called "ball-and-stick" language of chemical atoms and bonds. Substructural units which the data indicate are necessary parts of the explanation are grouped together as "superatoms." Other constraints for good and bad arrangements of atoms (and superatoms) are specified on lists known as GOODLIST and BADLIST, respectively.[5]

CONGEN produces a complete and nonredundant list of molecular structures containing exactly the specified atoms and satisfying the

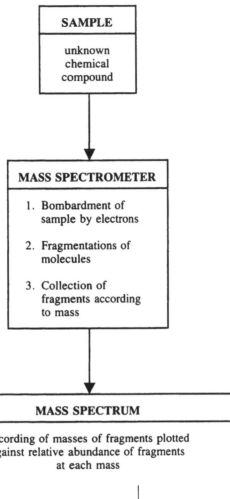

Figure 1. Data to Be Explained

specified constraints. Of the enormously large numbers of chemical structures with a specified atomic composition, the generator avoids constructing any that fail to contain the superatoms and prunes whole classes of structures (before instantiation) with respect to GOODLIST, BADLIST, and the other constraints.

Although the generator is mathematically complex, the underlying principle is to break the large generation problem into discrete steps and build progressively larger hypotheses at each step. Thus at various stages of the generation process, different heuristics can prune whole classes of partially specified hypotheses.

The unconstrained algorithm has been proved to produce all possible chemical graphs with a specified composition, without duplication [1]. Since there are hundreds of possibilities for six-atom structures, thousands for 7–8 atoms, millions and tens of millions for 15–20 atoms, the generator cannot profitably examine every possible explanation. The need for constraints is obvious, as is the need for a machine to carry out the generation and systematic exclusion of hypotheses.

CONGEN has been used as an aid to discovery by many chemists around the world. It is not without limitations, which are largely due to restrictions imposed by the ball-and-stick language.[6] However, the constraints are well enough understood to allow chemists to use this tool effectively [3].

Meta-DENDRAL

The Meta-DENDRAL program [4] is designed to aid chemists find and explain regularities in a collection of data. The hypotheses it formulates are general rules that explain the observed regularities. This activity is close to what most of us would call the "essence" of science, for it involves classifying phenomena as well as noticing regularities and discovering universal generalizations about them. Although the most revolutionary discoveries involve postulating new theoretical entities (i.e., developing a new theory), finding general rules is also a creative activity within an existing theory. It is at this level of scientific activity that the Meta-DENDRAL program operates. It does not postulate new terms but tries to find new regularities and explain them with rules written in the predefined vocabulary.

The "observations" the program starts with are empirical data collected on several known chemical compounds. The data have been

1. chemical composition of unknown sample:

   $C_{18}H_{24}O_2$

2. Specify constraints:

   (a) estrogenic steroid skeleton

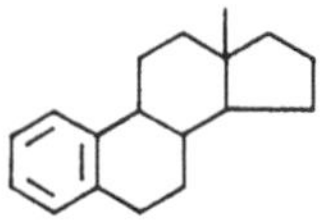

   (b) 2 hydroxyl groups [−OH]

   (c) one hydroxyl on aromatic ring

   (d) one hydroxyl on five-membered ring

3. Generate structural hypotheses with additional constraints that

   (3a) the hydroxyl in the aromatic ring is *not* adjacent to a ring juncture

   (3b) the hydroxyl in the 5-membered ring *is* adjacent to the quaternary carbon atom (i.e., carbon with 4 non-hydrogen neighbors)

4. Generated candidates =

   H1: 2-hydroxy-estradiol

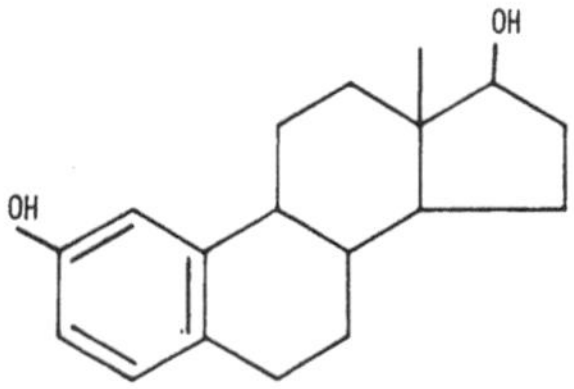

   H2: 3-hydroxy-estradiol

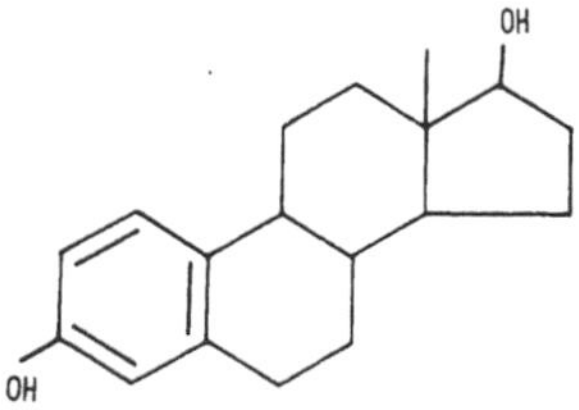

5. Rank hypotheses using the heuristic that the preferred position for hydroxyls in estrogenic steroids is that shown in H2.

   most plausible hypothesis = H2

   Figure 2. Simplified Structure Elucidation Example

limited to data from one commonly used analytical instrument, a mass spectrometer (described above). The regularities that the program can find are common modes of fragmentation and rearrangement of the known structures in the mass spectrometer. And the explanations of those regularities that it can discover are general rules causally relating "essential" features of molecules to their fragmentation behavior in the instrument (see figure 3).

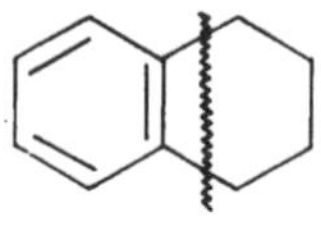

R1: If there is an aromatic ring joined to another
ring, break the second ring at the ring
junctures.

Figure 3. Example of a General Rule Explaining
Part of the Collection of Data

The fixed vocabulary of the theory is known to the program, as are criteria for allowable extension to the theory. A rule describes a general configuration of atoms around bonds that makes those bonds less stable under high-energy electron bombardment of the molecules in the mass spectrometer. The program emulates many of the reasoning aspects of manual approaches to rule discovery. It reasons symbolically, using a modest amount of chemical knowledge. It decides which data points are important and looks for fragmentation processes that will explain them. Then, as a chemist does, the program tests and modifies the rules.

Finding Regularities

The program first looks for regularities in the mass-spectrometric behavior of the given molecules.[7] Each data point is associated with the possible fragmentation processes that could have produced that datum within the mass spectrometer. Then the fragmentation processes for which there is substantial evidence are postulated as empirical regularities in the observed behavior of the given molecules. This part of the program is called INTSUM, for interpretation and summary of the data.

The INTSUM task is very much what Whewell called "colligation of facts," in which observations are gathered and interpreted [7]. Whewell noticed that interpretation of facts depends on an observation language whose legitimacy is supported by a theory, that fact gathering and theory building go hand in hand.

For each molecule in a given set, INTSUM first produces the plausible bond-cleavage processes that might occur, that is, breaks and combinations of breaks, with and without transfer of hydrogens and other neutral species. These processes are associated with specific bonds in a portion of molecular structure, or skeleton, that is chosen because it is common to the molecules in a given set. Then INTSUM examines the mass spectra of the molecules looking for evidence (spectral peaks) for each process. INTSUM gives explanations of spectral peaks for each molecule and then produces a summary showing the total evidence associated with each possible process.

Generating Explanatory Rules

The program next looks for rules to explain the regularities by searching a space of possible rules in much the same way that Heuristic DENDRAL searches its space of possible molecular structures to find an explanation of observed data. Whole classes of rules are avoided if all of their instances would fail to meet syntactic and evidential criteria of rulehood, thus constraining the search to a small fraction of the total space.

The form of any rule is a conditional sentence relating the subgraph environments of chemical bonds with fragmentations involving these bonds. For example, one well-known rule (which the program also rediscovered) is that the presence of a nitrogen atom in the environment of a carbon atom causes the C-N bond to cleave in the mass spectrometer, regardless of the other attachments of the atoms. The program found the rule in this example after noticing that in a dozen nitrogen-containing molecules there was substantial evidence associated with the cleavage of every C-N bond. Although many of the data points could be explained in other ways, this rule was preferred for reasons of simplicity and total evidential support. Occam's razor argues for dropping the redundant explanatory rules.

We used heuristic search to examine possible generalizations of the environments, where each generalization can be interpreted as a possible rule when coupled with information about the bond cleavages and transfers of hydrogens or other neutral species. Conceptually, the generator begins with the most general subgraph description R*R (where R is any unspecified atom and where the asterisk is used to indicate the bond cleaved, with the charged fragment written to the left of the asterisk). Then it generates refined descriptions by successively specifying one additional feature, in all possible ways. Currently we describe bond environments in terms of a topological, or connectivity, model of structure within the ball-and-stick language. We specify atom type, degree of substitution, number of hydrogen neighbors, or number of multiple bonds at any atom place. Other features of atoms can also be used if they are computable from the connectivity-graph model of a molecule—for example, ring size or chain length. But this is the current vocabulary in terms of which rules are written. The most useful rules lie somewhere between the overly general environment R*R and the overly specific complete bond-environment descriptions for a whole molecule.

The program continues to make rules more specific until it finds a daughter rule that is (a) specific enough to focus on one type of process (and to avoid many potential counterexamples) and (b) general enough to account for more than a few special cases.

Modifying Rules

The last phase of the program (RULEMOD) evaluates the plausible rules generated by RULEGEN and modifies them by making them more general or more specific. Its task is to analyze the validity of predictions made by the rules on the original set of molecules, modify the subgraph descriptions of the rules to improve the accuracy of their predictions, merge similar rules, and finally select a subset of the modified rules. RULEMOD will typically turn out a set of eight to twelve rules covering substantially the same data points as an original set of approximately twenty-five to one hundred rules, but with fewer incorrect predictions. The modification step is necessary after generation because, for efficiency reasons, not all the criteria of plausibility were used as constraints during generation. The local evaluation in RULEGEN has not discovered that different RULEGEN pathways may yield rules that are different but explain many of the same data points. Thus there is often a high degree of overlap in those rules generated by RULEGEN. Rules may have many counterexamples because this expensive test is also not made during generation. The scoring function used to discard implausible rules and rank the plausible ones captures the following intuitions:

(a) The score should reflect the strength of evidence, that is, it should be proportional to average peak intensity.
(b) Data points (peaks) that are uniquely explained by a rule should count more than peaks that can be explained by two or more rules.
(c) Negative evidence (peaks predicted and not found) should count heavily against a rule.
(d) Since the number of molecules in the set remains the same during rule formation and we insure that every rule applies to a minimum number of molecules (in our case, half the molecules), the score for purposes of selection need not explicitly consider the sample size. When we want to compare sets of rules formed from different sets of molecules, however, it will be necessary to weight the scores of rules by the number of molecules considered.

We have shown that the Meta-DENDRAL program is capable of rationalizing the mass-spectral fragmentations of sets of molecules in terms of substructural features of the molecules. On known test cases, aliphatic amines and estrogenic steroids, the Meta-DENDRAL program rediscovered the well-characterized fragmentation processes reported in the literature. On the three classes of ketoandrostanes for which no general class rules had previously been reported, the mono-, di-, and triketoandrostanes, the program found general rules describing the mass-spectrometric behavior of those classes [5]. This is the first instance we know of in which general symbolic laws have been discovered by a computer program and published in a scientific journal as new results.

Programs with knowledge of the scientific domain can provide "smart" assistance to working scientists, as shown by the reasoned suggestions this program makes about extensions to mass-spectrometry theory. We are aware that the program is not discovering a new framework for mass-spectrometry theory; to the contrary, it comes close to capturing in a computer program all we could discern by observing human problem-solving behavior. It is intended to relieve chemists of the need to exercise their personal heuristics over and over again, and thus we believe it can aid chemists in suggesting more novel extensions of existing theory.

MOLGEN

The MOLGEN computer program[8] is a third program we are building at Stanford. As of this writing (1978), it is still under development and is newer than DENDRAL and Meta-DENDRAL, so it will be described only briefly. The intent of MOLGEN is to put as much knowledge of molecular biology into a computer program as we need in order to provide intelligent assistance to working scientists. We are focusing on the knowledge used by faculty and staff in the Department of Genetics at Stanford in designing and debugging experiments with DNA. The *experiments* are of two major classes: structural analysis of DNA segments, and synthesis of new DNA segments with specified features.

The techniques for manipulating DNA segments must be described to the program: there are enzymes that cut and join as well as chemical and physical techniques. The knowledge base is stored as a hierarchy of concepts with many features associated with each concept. For example, under the concept CUTTING TECHNIQUES will be found NUCLEASE (i.e., an enzyme that breaks chemical bonds in the DNA backbone), and under that will be found ENDONUCLEASE and EXONUCLEASE. One of the site-specific ENDONUCLEASES is Eco-R1, a particular enzyme isolated from E.coli that cleaves DNA in specific places. Associated with the name of the particular enzyme will be a definition of its recognition site and a specification of experimental conditions under which the enzyme will work, such as the optimal pH range.

In designing experiments, the program is strongly driven by the goal as specified by the geneticist. The key to its operation is *systematic generation of plausible experimental plans*. It starts from an abstract description of the goal and successively refines the description in all plausible ways. For example, a synthesis experiment often involves implanting one DNA segment inside a larger DNA molecule. One of the abstract concepts involved in implantation is cutting; then one way of cutting is by using a nuclease, and so on until one of the particular steps is described as mixing the DNA with the cutting enzyme Eco-R1 under specified conditions.

The program may be able to propose novel experiments for the following three reasons:

(1) The knowledge base may eventually contain specific knowledge about *different* techniques or materials that are not known by the *same* human scientist.
(2) The *combinatorics* of applying one technique after another get to be more complex than humans can cope with.
(3) The program will be free to explore alternatives to the published methods that human scientists come to rely on heavily. The stereotypical experimental steps are handy mnemonic devices for humans, but they may also keep a person from seeing something novel. While MOLGEN's proposals themselves are built from unknown techniques, its sense of "combinatorial play" need not be restrained by stereotypes.

MOLGEN uses a large knowledge base of facts, associations, and heuristics to define the space of plausible sequences of experimental steps. Although the total space is immense, the reasoning program is guided by knowledge of plausible abstract plans and plausible refinements of those. The final hypothesis, then, is a detailed description of an experiment that achieves the goal, within a specified language of laboratory objects and procedures. The program is beginning to be used by molecular biologists, but without conclusive results at this time.

Limitations of the Heuristic Search Method

The major limitation of the heuristic search method in any domain is the necessity of finding (or inventing) a generator of possible solutions. In the case of molecular structures, finding the generating algorithm took many years. Lederberg's notational algorithm for unringed graph structures (described in [2]) was mapped into a generating algorithm with little difficulty, but the symmetries of cyclic graphs complicated the generation problem immensely. Not until considerable mathematical expertise had been focused on the problem was a generator invented that carried guarantees of complete and nonredundant generation. In the rule-formation domain, that means that we needed to invent a program that generates possible rules. That, in turn, required a strict definition of the allowable forms of the rules and a definition of the allowable primitive terms that add content to the form. The representation we have found for expressing rules is fixed for any one run of the program but can, at least, be modified or extended manually between runs.

A second major limitation on heuristic search is the necessity of finding heuristics, or rules of thumb, that guide the generator and constrain it from producing all syntactically allowable hypotheses. For rule generation it was necessary to find heuristics that steer the generator *toward* the small number of interesting rules and away from the very large number of uninteresting rules. The problem is that it is difficult to find these guiding principles. In addition, putting confidence in the heuristics requires an act of faith. Once that step is made, however, there is often the temptation to put too much faith in the heuristics and forget that the solutions were found in the context of a large number of assumptions. For example, one might tend to forget the criteria for data filtering, or the restrictions on how complex the hypotheses were allowed to become, or the criteria for excluding implausible hypotheses, or the limitations of the conceptual framework.

On the other hand, the *strengths* of the method should be equally obvious:

(1) We can guarantee that all implausible hypotheses have been excluded and that the remaining hypotheses are all the plausible ones. (The guarantee holds only within the conceptual frame defined for the program but is good for the life of that framework.)

(2) We can encode a scientist's incomplete and uncertain knowledge of the domain to help define the criteria of plausibility. The programs can be given these items in many levels of certitude—from those most central to the paradigm to those that are little more than ephemeral intuitions.

SUMMARY AND CONCLUSIONS

The traditional problem of finding an effective method for formulating true hypotheses that best explain phenomena has been transformed into finding heuristic methods that generate plausible explanations. The problem of giving rules for producing true scientific statements has been replaced by the problem of finding efficient heuristic rules for culling the reasonable candidates for an explanation from an appropriate set of possible candidates.

In the most creative heights of science, hypothesis formation is farthest from the "reach of method," as Whcwell says. But within the comfort of an established scientific theory, paradigm, or conceptual scheme, hypothesis formation usually does not involve the introduction of new concepts. The concepts are given and the task of a logic of discovery is to show how hypotheses should be formulated in terms of these concepts. Depending on the purposes at hand, and in part upon the science, the hypothesis may either *explain* a puzzling phenomenon (or set of phenomena) or *describe* objects and events within the scope of the science.

The problems with formulating this kind of logic of discovery are both difficult and numerous. Before any methods, heuristic or otherwise, can be given for "discovering" explanations or regularities, precise criteria of success for the logic must be formulated. When such criteria are clarified and refined for the specific science considered, then the methods could be said to succeed when they produce hypotheses that meet the criteria. The methods themselves will also be difficult to formulate in specific instances because of the difficulties in understanding the problem, representing the space of possible solutions, dividing the task into subproblems, and planning a solution, to mention the outstanding ones.

To a modest degree, the Heuristic DENDRAL, Meta-DENDRAL, and MOLGEN programs capture many of the notions of a logic of discovery. They are more systematic and less random than we have come to expect of creative guessers in science, but their methods are also more teachable and their results more reproducible.

NOTES

1. In addition, I owe a considerable debt to colleagues and friends at Stanford who helped shape these ideas, Professors E. A. Feigenbaum and J. Lederberg in particular.

2. For more information on heuristic search and other symbolic computation techniques, see [23].

3. Design issues for this program, and similar programs, are discussed in [9].

4. It is common practice to consult libraries of data associated with known compounds in order to find the best library entry that explains one's present set of data. The DENDRAL programs, however, are meant to discover explanations even when the data have not been previously recorded in a library.

5. Note that the source of these constraints has deliberately been left unspecified. In other publications [19] we describe a problem-solving program whose task it is to infer constraints from mass-spectrometry data. However, CONGEN does not know where the constraints come from, and most of the time chemists are much better at making these inferences from their data than the program is anyway.

6. For example, the program knows nothing of polymers, it knows nothing of bond angles or lengths, and it is limited in practice to structures containing 50–100 atoms.

7. The regularities in the data points themselves can be found by statistical pattern recognition programs and used to help interpret new data [24]. This, however, is not the approach used here, since we are looking for relations that provide some deeper insights into the theory of mass spectrometry.

8. MOLGEN has been implemented largely by M. Stefik and P. Friedland. See [14] for details.

REFERENCES

[1] Brown, H., and L. Masinter. 1974. An algorithm for the construction of the graphs of organic molecules. *Discrete Mathematics* 8:227.

[2] Buchanan, B. G., A. M. Duffield, and A. V. Robertson. 1971. An application of artificial intelligence to the interpretation of mass spectra. In *Mass spectrometry techniques and applications*, ed. G. W. A. Milne. New York: Wiley.

[3] Buchanan, B. G., and E. A. Feigenbaum. 1978. DENDRAL and Meta-DENDRAL: Their application dimension. *Artificial Intelligence* 11:5.

[4] Buchanan, B. G., and Tom Mitchell. 1978. Model-directed learning of production rules. In *Pattern-directed inference systems*, ed. D. A. Waterman and F. Hayes-Roth. New York: Academic Press.

[5] Buchanan, B. G., D. H. Smith, W. C. White, R. J. Gritter, E. A. Feigenbaum, J. Lederberg, and Carl Djerassi. 1976. Application of artificial intelligence for chemical inference XXII: Automatic rule formation in mass spectrometry by means of the Meta-DENDRAL program. *Journal of the American Chemical Society* 98–6168.

[6] Budzikiewicz, H., C. Djerassi, and D. H. Williams. 1967. *Mass spectrometry of organic compounds*. San Francisco: Holden-Day.

[7] Butts, Robert E. 1973. Whewell's logic of induction. In [11].

[8] Carhart, R. E., D. H. Smith, H. Brown, and C. Djerassi. 1975. *Journal of the American Chemical Society* 97:5755.

[9] Churchman, C. W., and B. G. Buchanan. 1969. On the design of inductive systems: some philosophical problems. *British Journal for the Philosophy of Science* 20:311.

[10] Feigenbaum, E. A., and J. Feldman, eds. 1963. *Computers and thought*. New York: McGraw-Hill.

[11] Giere, R. N., and R. S. Westfall, eds. 1973. *Foundations of scientific method: The nineteenth century*. Bloomington: Indiana University Press.

[12] Laudan, Laurens. 1973. Peirce and the trivialization of the self-correcting thesis. In [11].

[13] Leeson, G. 1977. A chat with Linus Pauling. *California Living* (section of the *San Francisco Sunday Examiner and Chronicle*), 17 July.

[14] Martin, N., P. Friedland, J. King, and M. J. Stefik. 1977. Knowledge base management for experiment planning. In *Proceedings of the Fifth IJCAI, Cambridge, Mass.*, 882. Pittsburgh: Dept. of Computer Science, Carnegie-Mellon Univ.

[15] Newell, A. 1963. GPS, a program that simulates human thought. In [10].

[16] Polya, G. 1948. *How to solve it*. Princeton, N.J.: Princeton University Press.

[17] Simon, Herbert A. 1973. Does scientific discovery have a logic? *Philosophy of Science* 40:471–480.

[18] Schaffner, K. 1974. Logic of discovery and justification in regulatory genetics. *Studies in History and Philosophy of Science* 4:349–385.

[19] Smith, D. H., B. G. Buchanan, R. S. Engelmore, A. Yeo Duffield, E. A. Feigenbaum, J. Lederberg, and C. Djerassi. 1972. Applications of artificial intelligence for chemical inference. VIII. An approach to the computer interpretation of the high resolution mass spectra of complex molecules. Structure elucidation of estrogenic steroids. *Journal of the American Chemical Society* 94:5962.

[20] Smith, D. H., B. G. Buchanan, R. S. Engelmore, H. Adlercreutz, and C. Djerassi. 1973. Applications of artificial intelligence for chemical inference. IX. Analysis of mixtures without prior separation as illustrated for estrogens. *Journal of the American Chemical Society* 95:6078.

[21] Smith, D. H., B. G. Buchanan, W. C. White, E. A. Feigenbaum, C. Djerassi, and J. Lederberg. 1973. Applications of artificial intelligence for chemical inference—X. INTSUM. A data interpretation and summary program applied to the collected mass spectra of estrogenic steroids. *Tetrahedron* 38:3117.

[22] Toulmin, S. E. 1961. *Foresight and understanding*. Bloomington: Indiana University Press.

[23] Winston, P. H. 1977. *Artificial intelligence*. Reading, Mass.: Addison-Wesley.

[24] Zander, G. S., and P. C. Jurs. 1975. *Anal. Chem.* 47:1562.

5

Thoughts on the Limitations of Discovery by Computer

Carl G. Hempel

INTRODUCTORY REMARKS

Some years ago, in a lecture I gave at the University of Pittsburgh, I remarked, somewhat incidentally, that there could be no general algorithmic rules of scientific discovery, that is, rules specifying a unique step-by-step procedure that would lead, from any given set of empirical data, to a general theory covering or explaining the data. For otherwise, I argued, those rules could be used to construct a general computer program for scientific discovery, such that if a computer equipped with it were given a list of data obtained by experiments involving precipitations, explosions, or changes of color, temperature, or mass of interacting substances, then it should be able to print out the atomic and molecular theory of matter, the theory of valence bonds, and so forth. But such a feat of discovery, I concluded, was impossible for a computer because the theory in question makes use of terms, such as *atom, molecule, valence bond,* and many others, which do not occur at all in the description of the experimental data given to the computer. What general mechanical rules of discovery could possibly yield the novel concepts required for the explanatory theory? This example seemed to me to illustrate the need, in scientific discovery, for a kind of creative imagination that cannot be matched by any computer.

In the ensuing discussion, a member of the audience objected that, after all, the human brain was a computer, and it clearly could generate such novel concepts and theories. The objector was Professor Herbert Simon, whom I first met on that occasion.

His counterargument might be said to beg the question; for it simply assumes that those structural and functional features which enable a brain to discover new theories are just those of a sophisticated computer. On the other hand, the conception of a computer presupposed in my argument is not very precise and is too narrow in at least one respect: computer programs need not be based exclusively on algorithmic rules; as Professor Simon pointed out to me, they may incorporate, for example, certain steps involving random procedures.

I do not think that the inclusion of this feature would enable a computer to make scientific discoveries in the grand manner envisaged in the example of the atomic and molecular theory of matter; but the specific computer achievements discussed at the present workshop certainly give impressive evidence that computers can indeed make important discoveries of certain kinds, and that in so doing they can outperform human investigators. I would like, therefore, on this occasion to offer some further tentative considerations on the reach of discovery by computer.

DISCOVERY OF DIAGNOSTIC HYPOTHESES
FOR INDIVIDUAL CASES

The principal aim of the programs considered at this workshop is the discovery of what I will call diagnostic hypotheses for individual cases. A hypothesis of this kind explains why some particular "case"—for example, a given animate or inanimate object—possesses a certain set of characteristics, described by a given body of data; and it does so by assigning the given particular case to a specific diagnostic class or category whose members possess the characteristics in question as well as other common features by reference to whose presence or absence in the given case a tentative diagnostic hypothesis may be subjected to further tests.

In the case of the INTERNIST program, the individual cases are patients exhibiting the symptoms described in the data; the diagnostic categories are various kinds of illness. For each of the diagnostic categories it provides for, the program contains a set of what might be called principles of manifestation; these specify for each of the disease categories a set of signs and symptoms by which the disease manifests itself. These principles of manifestation may be regarded as providing operational criteria of application for the diagnostic categories; they have the character of empirical laws of strictly universal or else of statistical form, asserting that all, or a specified percentage, of the cases falling into a diagnostic category C display a certain symptom S.

On the basis of the principles of manifestation and of heuristic procedural rules built into it, the program constructs, for symptomatic data fed into the computer, tentative diagnostic hypotheses for the individual case to which the data pertain. Such hypotheses might roughly be said to explain the given symptoms to the extent that the diagnostic category specified by the hypothesis calls for the presence of those symptoms. Failure of an acceptable diagnostic hypothesis to account for some of the given symptoms is a possibility explicitly countenanced by the "Disregarding" clause permitted in the final diagnosis.

The DENDRAL program is designed to discover, or to diagnose, the molecular structure of a given organic compound on the basis of symptomatic data obtained by mass-spectrometric analysis of that compound. Again, the program includes principles of manifestation; these associate specific mass-spectrometric findings with particular molecular structures and thus make it possible to explain the spectrometric findings for a given substance by a diagnostic hypothesis assigning to that substance a certain molecular structure.

The search for an optimal explanatory hypothesis might proceed, "in principle," by systematically constructing all possible diagnostic hypotheses for the given case and testing them by reference to the data; actually, such a procedure would be immensely inefficient and practically inapplicable in all cases of scientific interest. The great value and distinction of the DENDRAL program lies in the fact that its search for suitable hypotheses is guided by a set of subtle and efficient heuristic principles, as explained in Bruce Buchanan's "Steps toward Mechanizing Discovery" (chapter 4 of this volume).

These sketchy and schematic observations have left unmentioned a variety of most ingenious features of the two programs referred to, and they have given no indication at all of the impressive successes of their actual applications. But I hope that these omissions will occasion no distortions in a few general considerations now to be outlined concerning the question of limitations of the discoveries that can be made in this way.

SOME LIMITATIONS OF DIAGNOSTIC COMPUTER PROGRAMS

The discoveries achievable by programs of the kind just considered are subject to various limitations, in particular (1) the limitation of all discoverable hypotheses to sentences expressible with the logical means of the given computer language; (2) limitation of the available vocabulary to one that is antecedently given and fixed; (3) limitations of the available principles of manifestation (more generally: limitations of the given empirical background assumptions).

As for the vocabulary, both the set of terms available for the description of the data and the set of terms available for the specification of diagnostic categories—and hence, of diagnostic hypotheses—are antecedently fixed. This makes it impossible for the computer to "discover" new signs and symptoms of a disease or to modify the system of its diagnostic categories by introducing additional ones or perhaps by partitioning available categories (e.g., by distinguishing several different types of pneumonia or of diabetes): the new vocabulary required for such purposes just is not available in the program.

Moreover, the discovery of new symptoms or new diagnostic categories would evidently require the establishment of new principles of manifestation; but that possibility is precluded by the fact that the set of all principles of manifestation available to the computer is antecedently fixed by the program.

The discoveries that can be made by means of the programs under consideration are arrived at, basically, by a skillful heuristic search in the fixed class of all the diagnostic hypotheses that can be expressed in the vocabulary of the program; this leads to the selection of a small subset of hypotheses which, in consideration of the given set of principles of manifestation, best explain the symptoms shown by a given case, as described in the given symptom-vocabulary of the program. But evidently there may be much better diagnostic-explanatory hypotheses for a given case which, however, the program cannot possibly discover because of the limitations just indicated.

The difficulties would remain unaffected if certain randomizing features were incorporated into the program. One way of doing this is described (and, in effect, rejected) in Buchanan's paper, "Steps towards Mechanizing Discovery": a computer might be programmed to generate hypotheses randomly, to test each of them by reference to the available evidence, and to stop when a hypothesis was found to be successful in explaining the evidence. Clearly, the vocabularies for the description of the evidence and for the random formulation of hypotheses would still be limited to those initially specified for the program.

DIFFICULTIES FOR THE DISCOVERY OF NEW DIAGNOSTIC PRINCIPLES AND OF THEORIES

The limitations just mentioned, which result from the fixity of the available principles of manifestation, can be overcome to some extent, however. The powers of a diagnostic computer program can surely be enhanced so as to permit the discovery of "new" principles of manifestation linking one of the available diagnostic categories, say C, to certain manifesting symptoms that can be described with the available symptom-vocabulary but that are not linked to C by any of the initially given principles of manifestation. To this end the computer might collect those cases which, by means of the initially given principles of manifestation, it had already diagnosed as instances of C, and it might then scrutinize them for further traits that are describable in the vocabulary of the program and that show a strong correlation with C. This procedure could lead to the discovery of new general principles of manifestation.

Meta-DENDRAL is a very sophisticated program aimed at the discovery of such general principles, or "rules," of manifestation (see, e.g., Bruce Buchanan, "Steps toward Mechanizing Discovery," cited above, and his account in "The DENDRAL Project: A Short Summary," HPP-77-17 Working Paper, Heuristic Programming Project, Computer Science Department, Stanford University). The rules, or general principles, however, that lend themselves to discovery in this manner are clearly limited to hypotheses that are expressible entirely in the given vocabulary of the program and with the logical means embodied in its language. But the formulation of powerful explanatory principles, and especially theories, normally involves the introduction of a novel conceptual and terminological apparatus. The explanation of combustion by the conflicting theories of dephlogistication and of oxidation illustrates the point.

The new concepts introduced by a theory of this kind cannot, as a rule, be defined by those previously available; they are characterized, rather, by means of a set of theoretical principles linking the new concepts to each other and to previously available concepts that serve to describe the phenomena to be explained. Thus the discovery of an explanatory theory for a given class of occurrences requires the introduction both of new theoretical terms and of new theoretical principles. It does not seem clear at all how a computer might be programmed to discover such powerful theories.

It was no doubt this kind of consideration that led Einstein to emphasize that there are no general systematic procedures which can lead the scientist from a set of data to a scientific theory, and that powerful theories are arrived at by the exercise of the scientist's free creative imagination.

THE NEED FOR CRITERIA OF PREFERENCE FOR COMPUTER PROGRAMS AIMED AT SCIENTIFIC DISCOVERIES

The preceding considerations have glossed over one further question that requires at least brief consideration. In examining the thesis that there are no general systematic rules leading from given data to suitable explanatory hypotheses or theories, we have not paid sufficient attention to the question of what requirements a "suitable" hypothesis should meet.

One initially plausible answer—one that largely informed the computer programs referred to earlier—is that an appropriate hypothesis should explain all or most of the given data. But this alone surely is not enough, for otherwise a satisfactory hypothesis for any given set of data could be constructed trivially by conjoining the data: from that conjunction any one of the given data would be deducible. What is wanted is evidently a hypothesis that goes beyond the data by yielding correct predictions for as yet unexamined occurrences.

But clearly it cannot be required of a "suitable" hypothesis that all the predictions it yields must be certain to be true: that there can be no guarantee of this kind for any hypothesis is the root of the problem of induction.

To put the point somewhat differently: given a set of data, it is always possible to formulate various different hypotheses that explain the data; but these hypotheses will not all be considered equally reasonable or appropriate. Through a given set of points representing associated values of two variables such as the temperature and the length of a given metal bar, many different curves can be drawn; they all cover the given data, but they are not regarded as representing equally acceptable explanatory and predictive hypotheses concerning the connection between the two variables. A computer program for the discovery of acceptable hypotheses would therefore have to include criteria of preference to govern the choice among different hypotheses each of which covers the available evidence. The "scoring function" for the Meta-DENDRAL program, as discussed in Buchanan's "Steps toward Mechanizing Discovery," would be an example.

There are, indeed, several such criteria of preference that are frequently invoked—among them, simplicity and large range of potential applicability—but these notions have not, so far, received a precise characterization. Moreover, as Kuhn's account of scientific revolutions has emphasized, there are further considerations that affect the choice among competing theories in science; but these are to some extent idiosyncratic, and no exact and generally acknowledged formulation of corresponding criteria is presently available or likely to be forthcoming.

CONCLUSION

It has sometimes been suggested that just as, with further advances in programming, chess-playing computers may eventually beat even the ablest chess master, so improved computers programmed to make scientific discoveries may do better than the ablest scientists.

The preceding considerations suggest that this assumption is questionable. Indeed, in discovering hypotheses that are expressible in a language with fixed logical structure and a fixed vocabulary, computers with an ingenious heuristic program, a large memory, high speed, and great reliability of performance will be able to outperform a scientist, and in some cases, no doubt, have already done so.

But when the search is aimed at comprehensive theories which require the introduction of a new vocabulary and the formulation of theoretical principles in terms of it, then it is not clear how a suitable computer program might be designed.

Second, in the area of theoretical discoveries, the idea of doing "better" than scientists would surely have to concern respects other than speed of constructing and rapidity and extent of testing a theory: it would have to refer to the appropriateness of the theories constructed. Arguments for the superiority of theories discovered by computers would therefore have to invoke criteria of evaluation or preference for alternative theories that might be proposed. Hence, if there are no unambiguous criteria of that kind, as has been suggested, then the claim that a computer program might lead to better theories than the efforts of human investigators would lack a clear meaning.

6

The Logic(s) of Evaluation in Basic and Clinical Science*

Henry E. Kyburg, Jr.

I

Let me begin with some general remarks on logic and evaluation. Logic is concerned with the evaluation of argument or inference. It may also be concerned with thinking processes or cognitive processes; but a logician can get a handle on these processes only when they are made publicly accessible in linguistic form or are embodied even more concretely in computer circuitry. Logic is what is involved when we argue from given premises to a conclusion, or, in a less obviously linguistic form, when we infer from given facts or bits of evidence to another fact or state of affairs or diagnosis. Even in the latter case, if the inference is to be publicly accessible and subject to interpersonal controls and objective evaluation, it must be capable of expression in linguistic form. I shall thus assume, henceforth, that we are considering arguments in a specified language, though I shall not assume that the language is fixed once and for all: to discover a new disease entity is to justify an expansion of our medical vocabulary.

Arguments (and hence logics) may be divided into (at least) two general categories: inductive and deductive. This is a classical distinction. Valid deductive arguments are those whose conclusions *must* be

*Research on which some of the material presented here is based has been supported by the National Science Foundation, to which gratitude is hereby expressed.

true if their premises are true. Good inductive arguments are those that confer credibility, or acceptability, or practical certainty on their conclusions.

Deductive logic is concerned with the standards for deductive argument. The paradigm is of course the logic of mathematical argument. Though the matter is more controversial than meets the eye, for present purposes I shall include set theory, and thus mathematics in general, as part of deductive logic. Thus the argument whose premise is that the side of a given Euclidean square is of length L and whose conclusion is that its area is L^2, I take to be deductive. On exactly the same grounds the argument whose premise is that 10% of the A's are B's and whose conclusion is that 90% of the A's are non-B's is to be construed as a deductive argument, subject to evaluation by well-understood principles of deductive logic. The so-called probability calculus is as much a part of mathematics as is linear algebra; the only question is whether or not the letter P that occurs in the characteristic axioms is given an interpretation that makes those axioms true. This is a significant point, since some philosophers and statisticians write as though the probability calculus were inductive logic. It is not. It is a matter of unadulterated deductive logic. Of course the letter P may be given an interpretation that makes those particular deductions of special interest in the evaluation of inductive arguments; but that is as true of algebra as of probability theory.

We can say that inductive logic is concerned with standards for inductive argument, but that doesn't get us very far. The moment we attempt to go further, we got bogged down in controversy—including controversy about whether there is any such thing as inductive logic. That particular controversy I shall leave to one side; it is perfectly clear that physicians and researchers offer arguments and make inferences that do not, cannot, and should not conform to the standards of deductive argument—that is, they offer arguments in which it is *possible* that the premises may be true and the conclusion false; and it is also perfectly clear that on an intuitive level we can distinguish between better and worse arguments of this sort. The controversial issue is whether it is possible to develop a *logic* of such arguments—that is, public and formal standards that can be used in evaluating them. I shall assume that it is possible, at least in some degree; to assume otherwise is to give up without trying.

We must nevertheless confess that if this part of logic started in the seventeenth century, it has not progressed much since. Deductive logic has been a perennial distraction to the investigator into scientific argument. Popper (1959) and Kuhn (1962) are arch anti-inductivists, and the general scheme of most diagnostic computer programs is Popperian: generate hypotheses and falsify them deductively. Such schemes are not taken literally: we all know that there are no error-free data and that therefore there can be no error-free rule for eliminating hypotheses. The scheme is frankly an idealization. But we may wonder if it represents the best, or most enlightening, or most useful, idealization.

To be sure, *some* data may be "practically certain." But in principle the elimination rules should allow for the reinstatement of rejected hypotheses. At base we are dealing with inductive arguments. This applies just as much to the logician's analysis of scientific argument as to AI computer programs and seems to me to entail no more insurmountable problems in the one case than in the other.

Most people who suppose that an inductive logic is possible suppose that it has something or other to do with probability in some sense or another. There is no widespread agreement on *what inductive logic is,* or on *the sense of probability involved,* or even on *how it is supposed to function.* In what follows I propose to offer some suggestions regarding these three questions, then to look at the bearing that these answers have on some very general epidemiological and clinical questions, and finally to turn to some relatively (but only relatively) concrete applications.

II

Let us begin by asking about the function of inductive logic. Inductive arguments exist; some are better than others; and we would like to be able to tell which are which. In particular, it is desirable to have some sort of framework, some sort of machinery, for resolving disagreements about inductive arguments. For example, consider an epidemiological study. It is alleged to lead to a certain conclusion. It is obvious that the conclusion is not a deductive consequence of the raw data alone. Much of what enters into the conclusion depends on previously established knowledge; a whole body of scientific knowledge concerning physics, chemistry, and psychology, as well as medicine, is presupposed. But the conclusion is not a deductive consequence of the combination of this body of knowledge with the raw data either. The argument is statistical in character. What is alleged is not that it is *impossible* that the conclusion be false while the data and the presupposed knowledge are true, but that the knowledge and the data render the conclusion *acceptable* or *highly probable*. Such arguments, as we all know from the newspapers and the erratic behavior of the FDA, are controversial. The epidemiological argument can be challenged in a number of ways: the statistical analysis is inappropriate; the controls are inadequate; the sampling is biased; the conclusion conflicts with a part of that very body of scientific knowledge which was presupposed; certain factors assumed to be independent are known not to be independent; and so on.

Sometimes these challenges can be overwhelming; everybody agrees (after the event) that the study was a poor one. Sometimes these challenges can be definitively answered. But quite often the matter remains controversial, not merely in that the conclusion receives the Scottish verdict "not proven" but in the sense that some people think that the challenges have undermined the study and others think that they have not. This is a question of logic and not a question of fact. What is at issue is the import of the *given* evidence, not whether *further evidence* or *another study* could give us more information. And this is important, because we must make decisions, both individual and social, on the basis of the evidence we have. We can always learn more by getting more evidence, but this is often neither feasible nor desirable. Gathering more evidence can be expensive in time, in money, and in human suffering.

It is precisely in this region of controversy that I take inductive logic to be of most immediate usefulness. It is also true, of course, that the more we understand about inductive logic, the more we are in a position to design our experiments and plan our studies in such a way that their results cannot be successfully challenged, except by new evidence.

If inductive logic is to provide a framework within which potential or actual disagreement can be resolved, we shall want it to be both general and objective. We want it to be general in the sense that the principles it embodies are to have very wide application, and nearly universal appeal. We cannot achieve strictly universal appeal, since there are individuals who are simply irrational in some respects. We do not let this sort of irrationality undermine our standards of deductive logic, and we should not worry about the lunatic fringe in this case either. We want our inductive logic to be objective in the sense that mathematics is objective: there is a general procedure by means of which disagreements about mathematical arguments can ordinarily be resolved. The steps in a mathematical proof can be expanded and filled out to whatever degree is needed to insure agreement. The same should ideally be true of our inductive logic. In the case of a controversial epidemiological study, it should be possible for the parties to the controversy to make the statistics more explicit and the contents of the assumed body of scientific knowledge more explicit, in such a way that they can eventually reach agreement on the cogency of the argument.

Note that in neither case could a sensible person demand that the argument be made wholly explicit from the outset. Mathematical "proofs" are not *proofs* in the sense of first-order logic; they are highly abbreviated, but they can be expanded as needed to approach a proof in strict sense. In inductive arguments, such a demand would be even more out of place, since one difference between an inductive argument and a deductive one is that an inductive argument can be undermined by the addition of a premise while a deductive one cannot. Thus a completely explicit inductive argument would have to specify the complete contents of the corpus of knowledge it is based on, and this would be a pointless task for a person, though formalization might make it relatively feasible for a computer.

Let us be just a shade more formal about all this. I have referred to a presupposed body of knowledge. Let us represent this by a set of statements K in a specified language. Let us represent the data of our inference by D, and our conclusion by C. What we are after are, as Pople (1975) puts it, "criteria . . . for deciding when the weight of the evidence is sufficient to permit reasonably confident judgments to be rendered." Put another way, we want criteria for deciding when C is acceptable, or practically certain, or probable enough, given the combination K_D of background knowledge K and data D.

Two very quick remarks: what counts as a great enough weight of evidence to permit confident judgments in one circumstance may not count as great enough in another circumstance; what is at stake bears on what constitutes "enough weight." Second, it should be obvious that "acceptability" is always tentative: C may be acceptable relative to the background knowledge K and the data D but no longer acceptable when either K or D is expanded. There is nothing irrevocable about acceptance.

I propose to interpret "sufficient weight of evidence" simply in terms of probability. The criterion for the acceptability of the conclusion C, given K and D, is simply that its probability be greater than .9, or .95, or .99, or .999—whatever is appropriate to represent "practical certainty" in a given circumstance. This, of course, depends on what is at stake, and that is a matter of ethics or value theory. I am not suggesting that the determination of what constitutes practical certainty in a given context is either easy or uninteresting; I am suggesting only that this question should be kept separate from the *logical* question of the degree to which given evidence supports a given conclusion. It is sometimes suggested that the two questions cannot be divided, and that the probability of a conclusion should somehow reflect its importance, and should be different in different situations, even when the evidence and the background knowledge are the same. My feeling is that utter confusion lies at the end of this route.

The interpretation of probability that allows for the objective evaluation of conclusions relative to both data and background knowledge in an explicit and objective way is the epistemological interpretation, developed in Kyburg 1974 and in Kyburg 1983. Since this interpretation is relatively unfamiliar, I must say something about it.

First, it is a logical interpretation: probability is defined for statements such as C, relative to sets of statements representing bodies of knowledge, such as K_D. Given a statement C and a set of statements K_D, the probability of C relative to K_D is determined.

Second, if two statements C and C^* are known to have the same truth value in K_D, they have the same probability. Two special cases may serve as illustration: if C and C^* are logically equivalent, they have the same probability relative to any body of knowledge K_D. If C and C^* both belong to the set of statements K_D, they have the same probability (the maximum probability) relative to K_D.

Third, probabilities are represented by subintervals of the interval $[0,1]$ rather than by points in that interval.

Fourth, every probability corresponds to a *known* relative frequency or measure in the following sense:

The probability of C relative to K_D is the interval (p, q) just in case:

(1) it is known in K_D that C has the same truth value as a statement of the form $\ulcorner x \in y \urcorner$;

(2) there is a class z such that, relative to K_D, x is a random member of z with respect to belonging to y;

(3) there is a statement in K_D to the effect that the proportion or frequency or measure of z's among y's falls in the interval (p,q), and this is the most informative statement we have about y's among z's.

Fifth, the notion of randomness just mentioned, like that of probability, is epistemological. The formal definition is too complicated to give here, but the idea behind the definition is that of choosing the right reference class. Or, as it has been put here, defining or choosing the right population. Here are simple illustrations of the two main principles behind the definition:

Suppose you are concerned with the probability that a given pregnancy, if allowed to go to term, will result in the birth of a child with a certain defect. You know that in the population in general, the frequency of live births exhibiting that defect is about one in ten thousand. You know that the mother had a full sister who exhibited that defect, and (on theoretical genetic grounds) that the frequency with which that defect occurs among live births to mothers who have full sisters exhibiting the defect is about one in ten. You also know, of course, that the particular embryo in question either has that defect or does not have it. If this represents the relevant body of knowledge, the appropriate probability is a tenth: not a ten-thousandth, since you have knowledge that puts the case in a smaller reference class in which the frequency of the defect differs. And not the whole interval $[0,1]$ (the frequency with which the embryo in question is *known* to suffer the defect), since there is a reference class that gives us more useful information than that.

Suppose that an individual comes from a community of individuals among which 10% have a history of disease D. The individual, being a foundling, does not know whether or not there is a history of D in his family. Half the foundlings come from families with a history of D. Among individuals with D the frequency of allergic reaction to treatment T is 0.7; among others the frequency of allergic reaction to T is 0.1. What are the chances that this individual will have an allergic reaction to T?

One might argue that in the population as a whole, the frequency of allergic reactions is $0.16 = .1 \times .7 + .9 \times .1$, and that therefore our patient has a probability of .16 of exhibiting the reaction in question. But this would be wrong, since half the foundlings come from families with a history of D. What we should instead consider is the ordered pair consisting of the individual *and* treatment, and use Bayes' theorem (*applied to known frequencies*) to yield the result that the treatment applied to that individual will generate an allergic reaction with probability $0.4 = \frac{1}{2} \times .7 + \frac{1}{2} \times .1$.

The former principle is the subset principle; the latter is the product-set principle.

More specific illustrations of the principles lying behind the formal definition of randomness will appear in due course.

III

One thorny nest of issues which arises in epidemiology as it does to some degree in many statistical inquiries concerns the question of randomization. Consider first the exhortation that in order for an inference to be properly based on a sample from a population, the sample must be a random one. In the context of this exhortation, what is generally intended is that the sample be selected from the population by a mechanism that will in the long run select each sample of the given size with equal frequency. Note, for example, the discomfort Nugent et al. (1964) seem to suffer with regard to the fact that this condition cannot generally be met for "prior" probabilities.

Suppose that we want to estimate the prevalence of a certain disease among a certain group of individuals. Suppose that there are N individuals in the group in question and that we are going to draw a sample of n of them. I shall argue that the random-sampling condition is neither necessary nor sufficient for the soundness of an inference from the frequency in the sample to an estimate of the frequency in the population.

The statistical basis for this inference is that practically all n-membered subsets of a population exhibit a prevalence very close to that in the population as a whole. This is simply a set-theoretical fact—a truth of logic, if you will. The equivalence we make use of is the mathematical truth that the prevalence in the population differs from the prevalence in the sample by less than ϵ if and only if the prevalence in the sample differs from that in the population by less than ϵ. If we know the frequency in the sample to be r, we need to satisfy only one more condition in order to say that it is practically certain that the prevalence in the population is $r \pm \epsilon$. That condition is that the sample be random in the epistemological sense. To spell that out a bit more for this case, what we require is that we have no grounds for placing that sample in a special subclass of the class of all n-membered subsets in which the frequency of representativeness is known to be rarer than it is in general. I shall distinguish between frequency or stochastic randomness (that with which the exhortation to sample in a certain way is concerned) and epistemological randomness, about which I have just been talking.

Let us first consider sufficiency. The argument behind the exhortation to obtain a sample that has frequency randomness is the following: If the sample is obtained by a mechanism that obtains each possible sample with equal frequency in the long run, it follows that the frequency with which representative samples are obtained by that mechanism is exactly the same as the frequency with which n-membered subsets of the population are representative. Thus if we follow the principle, we can be sure that *in the long run* we will be practically always correct in our estimate, since practically all the subsets of the population are representative.

But let us distinguish two cases: the predata case and the postdata case. Before we have obtained our sample, the argument for frequency randomness does provide a sufficient condition for the acceptability of the conclusion that the frequency in the sample *will* be about the same as the frequency in the population. While this is true, it provides us with no information, since, not having drawn the sample, we do not know what the frequency in the sample is. No substantive conclusion concerning the frequency of the disease in the population is possible.

Now consider the postdata case. We have drawn our sample, let us say, by an appropriate mechanism that provides a stochastically random sample. We consider two subcases. Either there is no sample that would be intuitively regarded (or regarded by the epistemological criterion) as inadequate or misleading for the inference in question, or there is such a sample. If there is no such sample, then again satisfaction of the frequency-randomization condition is sufficient for the cogency of the argument—but it is so only because *any* sample would be adequate; this is an uninteresting case. The interesting case is that in which some sample of n would be regarded as not forming a good basis for the inference to the prevalence of the disease in the population. For example, the population may contain both men and women, members of various races, individuals of various ages. A sample consisting only of white girls between the ages of fourteen and sixteen would be regarded as a poor basis for the inference in question, on the very sound ground that we know that many diseases exhibit different frequencies among men and among women, among individuals of different ages, among individuals of different races. (I leave to one side the possibility of stratified sampling; precisely the same issues can be raised there as I am raising here for simple random sampling.) If this sample is a poor one for the purpose of inference, frequency randomization is not sufficient for the soundness of the subsequent inference: in the long run, given satisfaction of the frequency-randomization condition, this sample will have to occur just as often as any other sample. When it does I shall use my common sense—or the epistemological notion of randomness—and select another sample.

What we have established is that in the interesting case—the case in which the sample has already been drawn, and in which there exist samples we would not be willing to use as a basis for inferring the prevalence of the disease in the population—frequency randomization is not sufficient for the cogency of the inference.

To establish that that condition is not necessary is even easier: Suppose there is some sample which, obtained by a method satisfying the frequency-randomization condition, would suffice as the basis for a cogent inference. That sample can also be selected by "arbitrary" or "haphazard" or "deliberate" methods that do not meet the condition. But the sample itself is the same sample, and if it suffices as a basis for inference in one case, it does so in another.

All of this is not to say that there is no place for randomization in experimental design. It has already been pointed out that in the predata analysis of experimental design, frequency randomization is sufficient to insure the high probability (still predata) that the sample *will* be representative. It is thus relevant to forming our expectations about what we may get out of an experiment or study. After the data are in, then it is no longer relevant: what counts then is the epistemological condition, for what we are concerned about is what we know about that particular sample we in fact have which may interfere with its soundness as a basis for inference.

More important, as anyone who has tried to do any actual sampling knows, to select deliberately a sample that does not exhibit some significant bias that you *should* have been able to guard against is very difficult indeed. One worries about whether there are too many of this sort of individual, or whether maybe such and such a sort is overrepresented, or whether there are not enough individuals of this other kind. Using a table of random numbers or some other mechanical device can save a lot of worry and thought. But in the final analysis, what we need to think about is not the frequency randomness of the mechanism by which we select the sample but the epistemological randomness of the sample we actually have *after* we have selected it.

The assessment of the inductive argument of a prevalence study requires that we focus on the epistemological probability of its conclusion. The claim is that this probability is high. This, in the framework I offer, amounts to the claim that a frequency in a certain class is high and that a certain object or sample is a random member of that class. In general the frequency assertion is not controversial; what is controversial is the claim concerning randomness. To say that the study is unsound is to say that there are good reasons for relating the probability in question to a frequency in a different reference class. To pursue the same illustration, if the sample of *n* consists entirely of white girls between the ages of fourteen and sixteen, it is to observe that the prevalence of the disease in the population as a whole is unlikely to be the same as that in the set of samples that consist of white girls between the ages of fourteen and sixteen. This fact is something we *know;* it is represented among those statements in K_D, our corpus of medical knowledge. We *know* that the sample is one that is homogeneous with respect to sex, age, and race; and we know that the proportion of such samples that are representative is not high.

Let us draw a more interesting illustration from a well-known book on testing statistical hypotheses (Lehman 1959, 189–191). Suppose that we are assessing the effectiveness of a certain drug in the treatment of a certain disease. The experimental material consists of $m + n$ patients. A group of $m + n$ patients are selected from a population; m will be controls. The data yielded by the experiment will consist of measurement $X_1, \ldots X_m, Y_1, \ldots Y_n$, where the X's are the values obtained from the controls. The i'th measurement can be considered as the sum of two components, U_i, a characteristic of the i'th patient, and V_i, a characteristic of the i'th treatment. We assume that the U's are a sample from a population which is normal with mean μ and variance σ_1^2, and that the first m V's are distributed normally with mean η and variance σ^2, and that the next n V's are a sample from a population which is normal with mean ξ and variance σ^2.

Lehman concludes that in the experiment so described it is "clearly impossible to distinguish between H (no effect) and the alternatives." But, according to him, we can save the situation "through the fundamental device of randomization." The reason is that the contribution u_i of the i'th patient to the measurement can have any value at all: the u's are completely arbitrary. We assign the patients to the treatments at random. The expected value of the contribution of the patient to the measurement is now the same for each measurement (since each patient has the same probability of being the subject of the i'th measurement); and thus any difference between the average X value and the average Y value can be put down to the effectiveness of the treatment.

Obviously this hocus-pocus does not give us any more information than we would have gotten from the same group of m control individuals and n treatment individuals had they been provided "haphazardly" or "arbitrarily" instead of "through the fundamental device of randomization." Of course there is a point to the device of randomization: it is a psychological aid that helps the optimistic investigator to avoid biasing the sample in his own favor, and the pessimistic investigator from biasing the sample against himself. But the important question from the point of view of inductive logic and epistemological probability concerns the sample we actually end up with. We require that the X and Y values we get be a random member of the set of such bodies of data with respect to indicating a difference between η and ξ, and that a high proportion of such bodies of data do indicate whether or not there is such a difference.

It is easy to see that frequency randomization cannot provide an answer to this problem. Suppose that there are just two patients and that U has a large variance relative to V. Then by randomizing we can be sure that the *expected* value for U will be the same for each patient; we can also be sure (ahead of time) that X will be much bigger than Y, or that Y will be much bigger than X; which is to say that we can be sure in advance that the drug will be either very effective or very deleterious. But this is silly. It is like this variant on Basu's story (Basu 1971) of how to weigh an elephant: To calculate the average weight of two elephants, you flip a coin and take the average weight to be that of the elephant indicated by the flip. Your estimate, in the long run, will average out just right, though in each case it will be foolishly wrong, if the elephants differ significantly in size.

IV

Let us turn to another major strand in the controversies concerning the analysis of experimental evidence. This is provided by the problem of using conditional probabilities to modify prior probabilities in the light of evidence through Bayes' theorem. An example of an approach along these lines is provided by the paper of Nugent et al. (1964); a more general example is provided by the paper of Engel et al. (1976). In order to deal with the problems raised by this approach, I must say something about conditional probabilities.

First it should be noted that in a sense epistemological probability is always conditional: the probability of a conclusion C is relative to (conditional on) a body of knowledge K augmented by a body of data D. In addition, epistemological probabilities are coherent—that is, conform to the probability calculus—in the sense that, given any finite algebra of statements A, there exists a belief function B such that B is a function from the elements of A to the real numbers in the interval $[0,1]$, B satisfies the axioms of the probability calculus, and for every statement S in A, $B(S)$ belongs to the interval representing the epistemological probability of S. But when conditionalization is added to coherence, things may go awry. In particular, we should distinguish between epistemological conditionalization: What would the probability of C be if one were to add the statement S to the body of knowledge K and the data D? and stochastic conditionalization: What is the measure of z in y given w? Sometimes—always in the case of gambling apparatus and the like—these two notions coincide. The epistemological probability that the next toss of this die will yield a 1, given that it yields an odd number, is a third, just as is the measure of the set of tosses yielding a 1, among those that yield an odd number. But there are special situations where the two notions do not coincide.

Example: that a coin is tossed once and lands heads does not alter the epistemological probability (relative to my body of knowledge) that it is two-headed; that it is two-headed profoundly alters the epistemological probability (relative to my body of knowledge) that it will land heads on the next toss. Yet stochastic conditionalization requires that one probability change if and only if the other does. The example is unpersuasive only because one wonders if the fact that the coin landed heads does perhaps, in a very tiny degree, alter the probability that I attribute to its being two-headed. But I think there are examples that cannot be accounted for this way.

If we abandon conditionalization for probability, what can we say about instances in which conditionalization seems to be relevant? A lot. Conditionalization applies automatically to relations among frequencies and among measures. There are all kinds of instances in which, the appropriate conditions of randomness having been met, a conditional probability is given by a conditional measure.

In particular, suppose that the probability of C relative to K_D is (p,q) because C is known (in K_D) to be equivalent to $\ulcorner x \in z \urcorner$, and x is a random member of z relative to K_D, and it is known in K_D that the proportion of y's that are z's is in the interval (p,q). Suppose that if we add C^* to D the result is K_{D*}, and suppose that relative to $K_{D*} x$ is a random member of $y \cap y^*$ with respect to z. The new measure of z serving as a basis for the probability of C will be the measure of z in $y \cap y^*$. And of course the conditional measure of z in $y \cap y^*$ will conform to the axioms of the probability calculus, including axioms about conditionality, simply because the axioms of the probability calculus are set-theoretical truths as applied to finite frequencies, and definitional truths as applied to measures.

Suppose, for example, that an individual (note that it is a specific individual, not an individual selected from a population by a randomizing device) appears with symptom S. We know that the proportion of individuals with symptom S who have disease D is .5 (say). There is a test we can apply: among the individuals with D, the result R will occur 80% of the time; among individuals who do not have D, R will occur only 10% of the time. We apply the test and get result R. Bayesian reconstruction: the probability that the individual has D is .5. The conditional probability that he has D, given that the test result is R, is $.4/.45 = (.5 \times .8)/(.5 \times .8 + .5 \times .1) = .89$. Epistemological reconstruction: Prior to the test, the individual is a random member of the set of people with symptom S. (He may or may not be, relative to our total body of knowledge; I am assuming that he is for the sake of the argument.) Among such people 50% have D. Therefore the probability, at that point, that he has D is .5. (This is a "prior" probability—but there is nothing subjective about it. We suppose it to be based on cogent epidemiological evidence.) We give him the test and obtain result R. Of those people who have symptom S, are given the test, and yield result R, the proportion who have the disease is (by the same calculation) .89. Relative to the corpus of knowledge I have *after* giving him this test, the individual may be a random member of that class of people. (He also may not be, since I may have learned other things about him meanwhile.) If he is, the new number, .89, will be the probability, relative to my new body of knowledge, that he has D. Note that there is no conditionalization of *probability* going on here—all the conditionalization concerns measures or frequencies.

The same thing is true in the program designed for diagnosing Cushing's syndrome (Nugent 1964), but here there are some interesting twists. The basic calculation yields the frequency with which individuals who are entered into the program and have such and such a combination of test results have Cushing's syndrome. This is in principle a perfectly straightforward calculation concerning frequencies that one would perform using Bayes' theorem. Hence, I suppose, why it is called a Bayesian program. But there is a great simplification of Bayes' theorem possible if certain events are independent of others, given the presence of the disease or the absence of the disease. (Obviously the manifestations will not be independent of each other in general: in general they will be positively linked through the disease.) The simplification is important in two ways, which are easily seen if we look at the statistical basis for the inference. Suppose one is taking account of ten manifestations; if one assumes that these manifestations are independent in the presence of the disease and independent in the absence of the disease, one has twenty items of statistical information to take account of; if one is not assuming that these manifestations are independent, there are 2^{10} or a thousand combinations of manifestations to take account of. The data base that would allow us to make an inference concerning the relative frequency of Cushing's syndrome in each of a thousand cells would obviously have to be enormous.

On the other hand, one cannot simply assume that manifestations are stochastically independent. So what the creators of the program did was to test for independence among the signs to drop from the program signs exhibiting dependence on other signs. This is a matter of throwing away a small amount of information to achieve a large amount of computational simplification. This, of course, is an anti-Bayesian move: we are applying a chi-square test at the 5% level; and then we are accepting into K, our body of background knowledge, the assumption that the signs that reveal no dependencies are independent. The truth of this assumption (or, more realistically, its approximate truth) is required for the Bayesian calculation that lies at the heart of the program. This is a combination of moves that is hard to justify or account for on either of the dominant approaches to statistics, the Bayesian approach and the testing-theory approach. It is nevertheless intuitively appealing, and perhaps could be accounted for by an epistemological approach that took account of inductive acceptance.

The relative frequencies that serve to provide the grist for the Bayesian mill of this program are those among a set of individuals in whom

Cushing's syndrome is suspected. Suppose that a physician is confronted with such an individual. The positive and negative signs are entered into the program; the program computes a number. This computed number is not the epistemological probability for the physician that that individual suffers from Cushing's syndrome. The number is the computed relative frequency (approximate and subject to various assumptions) with which individuals exhibiting that complex of signs suffer from the disease. This frequency is an epistemological probability for the computer, since that the individual exhibits that complex of signs is all the relevant data the computer has concerning him. But whether or not the frequency represents an epistemological probability for the physician is another matter.

According to the characterization of epistemological probability I gave earlier, this frequency will yield an epistemological probability for the physician just in case the individual in question is a random member of the set of individuals exhibiting the complex of signs in question, with respect to suffering from Cushing's syndrome, relative to the corpus of knowledge of the physician. Since the physician knows a lot of things that the computer does not, this is open to question. This does not mean that it is open to whimsical or arbitrary question. If, relative to the physician's body of knowledge, the individual is not a random member of the class in question with respect to suffering from the disease, it can only be because that knowledge allows him to be placed in some *more appropriate* reference class. Two extreme cases are obvious: the physician may have the results of definitive tests and so may be in a position to assign an epistemological probability of 1 or 0 to the proposition that the patient suffers from the disease.

Less extreme cases are mentioned in the paper under discussion: the results of critical tests such as adrenal suppression or the determination of cortisol production can put the individual in a reference class in which the relevant frequency is significantly closer to 1 or 0; if those data are part of the physician's body of knowledge, the individual is not a random member of the set of individuals exhibiting the complex of signs he exhibits, relative to the corpus of the physician.

V

DIALOG (Pople, Myers, and Miller 1975), later known as INTERNIST and now as CADUCEUS, raises a number of interesting questions and issues on which the approach I have outlined may shed some light. What I wish to focus on are the three important functions, *Evokes*, *Manifests* (or *Frequency*), and *Import*.

Manifests is clearly intended to be a straightforward statistical function: *MANIFESTS(D,M)* is "an estimate of $F(M,D)$, the frequency with which patients with proven diagnosis D will display M as a manifestation of that disease" (p. 850). This is measured only on a scale from 1 (rarely) to 5 (always), but one may suppose that this is a reflection of the fact that one does not generally have precise knowledge of the frequency in question.

It should be noted that this association is a result of statistical or inductive inference; and we might as well interpret $F(M,D)$ as the frequency with which individuals with the disease D exhibit manifestation M, whether or not the diagnosis of D has been made or even considered. The *data* on which this knowledge is based consist of individuals with a "proven" diagnosis of D, and the frequency with which they exhibit M. On the basis of these data we may accept a generalization to the effect that individuals with D rarely, sometimes, . . . always, exhibit M. It is questionable whether anything would be gained by replacing the measures 1 through 5 by more explicit measures (between 0 and 10% of the time, between 10 and 20% of the time, etc., corresponding to the intervals in ordinary statistical hypotheses). One might in fact prefer to use intervals in order to reflect the amount of data on which the estimate is based. "Between 0 and 10%" requires more data than "Between 0 and 50%." In any case, there is an inductive step involved in incorporating these measures of association in the program.

It is noteworthy that there is no suggestion that this frequency enters directly into any sort of Bayesian computation.

By contrast with *Manifests*, *Evokes* is not suggested as a statistical function: it is construed as "an estimate of $L(D,M)$: the likelihood that if manifestation M is observed in a patient, disease D is its cause." These estimates are given on a six-point scale, 0 indicating that the manifestation is too nonspecific to draw any diagnostic conclusions, and 5 indicating that M is pathognomonic for D. There may be many ways of construing *likelihood* here, but it seems fairly clear that no construal should be allowed to conflict with known frequencies. If it is known, for example, that over 90% of the people with manifestation M have disease D, one would not want $L(D,M)$ to be low.

One can imagine two motivations for the lack of any talk of frequencies here. The first, of course, is that, as in the case of the function

Manifests, we may well not have enough statistical data to do more than classify the value of the function as "rare" or "frequent"—hence the desirability of using a six-point scale rather than point estimates of the frequency. The second is different. Physicians are presented with a sample of those who have the disease, and though there may or may not be statistical study of the frequency with which those who have *D* exhibit *M*, at least the data for such a study are available. But it is hard to imagine anyone making a serious attempt to sample the population of individuals who manifest "headache," say, and then to estimate the frequencies of various diseases in that population. So not only do we not have very good frequency data for evaluating *Evokes*, but we seem to have little motivation for getting that sort of data.

On the other hand, programs such as INTERNIST may provide such motivation. It could be, at least with regard to some manifestations, that better data concerning the frequencies with which people having those manifestations have various diseases would so greatly improve the accuracy of the program as to be worth obtaining, even though the data contribute only to the diagnostic process. I do not know whether or not this is true, but it seems to me at least a live possibility.

The *Import* of a manifestation is a measure (on a scale from 1 to 5) of "how readily an observed manifestation can be ignored" (p. 850). The intuitive idea seems to be that a manifestation of low import is relatively easy to explain away without invoking the disease in question, while a manifestation of high import should be explained by the disease model in question, since it is hard to explain away. Note that although *Import* is introduced as a one-place function on manifestations, its *use* in the second phase of the program is relativized to models: "counting against a model are . . . data not explained [by a model, which] are weighed in proportion to their import" (p. 851). This use of *Import* suggests that frequencies are not irrelevant to import value; we might, for example, construe *Import* as the frequency with which a manifestation is exhibited in cases of diseases *other* than the one under consideration.

The point of these remarks is not to suggest improvements in INTERNIST, nor even to indicate its possible inductive shortcomings. It is rather to suggest that even though the description of the system makes relatively little explicit mention of frequencies, the compelling import of the inductive part of the program lies in associations measured by known frequencies, where of course we are regarding a frequency as "known" even when it is known only very roughly. But it lies not in these frequencies alone but also in an epistemological condition; loosely speaking, the program may compute that 95% of individuals with the complex of manifestations given have disease D; in order to pass from this statement to the conclusion that Alice Jones suffers from D requires that she be considered a random instance of individuals with that complex of manifestations relative to what the computer knows. In order for *us* to come to the same conclusion she must be a random member of that set relative to what *we* know, and we should not lose sight of the fact that there are things that we can know that the program does not know.

VI

The two sorts of logic involved in basic and clinical science are inductive and deductive, and they are both involved in each. The deductive logic involved is the most straightforward and classical sort of deductive logic; it includes set theory and mathematics, of course, and thus the theory of measure and integration. Finite relative frequencies provably satisfy the axioms of the so-called probability calculus; beyond this there are plenty of acceptable empirical theories that involve measures satisfying the axioms of the probability calculus. But in medical science there are relatively few such theories; we are concerned primarily with approximate relative frequencies in finite classes. The logic of arguments involving such approximate relative frequencies is just the logic of mathematical argument. No new and special conditions concerning probability or randomness need be invoked at this level.

There is more to deductive logic than is called upon in the evaluation of mathematical argument. There are a variety of intensional logics: temporal logic, logics of belief and knowledge, deontic logic, causal logic, and so on. I have offered a way of looking at arguments in basic and clinical science which does not involve any of these esoteric logics. It involves the representation of a body of knowledge by a set of statements, or by a program in a computer, or by a combination of the two. These statements are straightforward extensional statements concerning individuals, more or less approximate relative frequencies with which individuals fall into various classes, more or less approximate distributions of quantities among sets of individuals, and the like. To the extent that stochastic conditionalization is important in arguments in either basic or clinical science, this conditionalization can be represented within these bodies of knowledge as conditional frequencies. All of this is in the realm of classical deductive logic.

But this logic is not enough for the evaluation of arguments in either basic or clinical science, since in either case the interesting conclusions we draw must go beyond what is deductively warranted by the evidence. Inductive logic is the logic required for the evaluation of strictly inconclusive, though perhaps overwhelming, argument. Statistical epidemiological arguments provide a paradigmatic instance of this sort of argument in basic science; diagnostic arguments provide a paradigmatic instance in clinical science. Both sorts of argument are controversial, sometimes, and in both kinds of instances the controversy stems from an incomplete understanding of inductive argument—that is, argument that leads from accepted premises to the acceptance of a conclusion warranted by high probability. To avoid confusion with other proposed interpretations of probability, I refer to this as epistemological probability.

Epistemological probability is defined in terms of known relative frequencies or measures (which may be known only very approximately) and an epistemological condition of randomness. Formulating this epistemological condition of randomness can be construed as formulating conditions for the correct choice of a reference class under certain epistemological circumstances. I have not characterized these conditions here, since they are somewhat complicated. But a constraint we impose on them is that the same probability be assigned to each of two statements known to have the same truth value. Note that the reference class may be a class of individuals, or of *n*-tuples of individuals, or of ordered pairs consisting of an individual and a class, or, in general, objects that are as complicated as you please. The result is that epistemological probability turns out to be a well-defined function from sets of statements representing bodies of knowledge and statements to intervals: given a body of knowledge and a statement, there is exactly one interval that represents the probability of that statement relative to that body of knowledge.

Given such a definition, we may construe most of the statistics of epidemiological arguments as relatively uncontroversial deductive manipulations. The potentially controversial step concerns the acceptability—that is, the high probability—of the conclusion, and this depends on the satisfaction of the relevant epistemological condition of randomness. For example, it may depend on whether, *after* we have selected a sample and examined its members, it is a random member of the set of equinumerous samples of the population in question with respect to revealing the incidence of a certain disease in that population. This is quite independent of the question of whether the sample is random in the stochastic sense of being obtained by a procedure with certain stochastic or long-run properties. A clear understanding of epistemological probability and epistemological randomness may well not eliminate controversy about epidemiological conclusions, but it can provide a framework in which argument and counterargument concerning whether given evidence warrants a given conclusion can progress toward resolution.

The problem of diagnosis is similar, in the sense that often the clinical data do not, even taken in conjunction with a body of medical knowledge, deductively imply that the individual in question has a certain disease. The conclusion, that the individual x has disease D, is only inductively warranted—that is, is warranted by high probability rather than by logical implication. As in the inferences of basic science, much of the argument is deductive and involves relative frequencies. This part of the argument can be extremely complicated, and enormous advantages can be gained by representing the relevant parts of medical knowledge in a computer program. But there is a final step that, as in epidemiology and generally in basic science, involves passing from high frequencies concerning a *class* of individuals to high probability or practical certainty regarding a *single* individual. This depends on an understanding of epistemological probability and epistemological randomness, and requires that we take account of all that we know, and not merely what is known or represented in the computer program or codified in textbooks. This is not a matter of intuition, though there may be room for that too in the decisions made by a physician, but of rational argument. The peculiarity of inductive logic is that the evaluation of an inductive argument requires attention to a whole body of knowledge. An increase in that body of knowledge may undermine the warrant for a probable conclusion as well as increase its warrant. There are always items of knowledge in the physician's rational corpus that are not represented in the text or the program, and these items may undermine or reinforce a particular conclusion concerning a particular individual, and may do so in a perfectly objective and rational way. But in order to judge whether or not they do so in a particular case, we must understand inductive logic, and particularly the central notion of epistemological randomness.

REFERENCES

Basu, D. 1971. An essay on the logical foundations of survey sampling. In *Foundations of statistical inference*, ed. V. P. Godambe and D. A. Scott. Toronto and Montreal: Holt, Rinehart & Winston.

Engel, Ralph L., et al. 1976. HEME: A computer aid to diagnosis of hematological disease. *Bulletin of the New York Academy of Medicine* 52:584–600.

Kuhn, Thomas S. 1962. *The structure of scientific revolutions*. Chicago: University of Chicago Press.

Kyburg, Henry E., Jr. 1974. *The logical foundations of statistical inference*. Dordrecht: Reidel.

———. 1983. The reference class. *Philosophy of Science* 50:374–397.

Lehman, E. L. 1959. *Testing statistical hypotheses*. New York: Wiley.

Nugent, Charles A., Homer R. Warner, John T. Dunn, Frank H. Tayler. 1964. Probability theory in the diagnosis of Cushing's syndrome. *Journal of Clinical Endocrinology* 24:621–627.

Pople, Harry E., Jr., Jack D. Myers, and A. Randolph Miller. 1975. DIALOG: A model of diagnostic logic for internal medicine. In *Advance Papers of the Fourth International Joint Conference on Artificial Intelligence, Tbilisi, Georgia, USSR*, 848–855. Cambridge, Mass.: Artificial Intelligence Laboratory, M.I.T.

Popper, Karl R. 1959. *The logic of scientific discovery*. London: Hutchinson Co.

7

More on the Logic(s) of Evaluation in Basic and Clinical Science

Teddy Seidenfeld

I would like to recognize and discuss two kinds of problems raised by Henry Kyburg in the preceding essay. First, we should note which issues are controversial only because of unsettled disputes among competing inductive logics. Second, we should become aware of which methodological challenges cut across the variety of inductive systems there are to choose from. As an illustration of the former problem I shall argue that questions about the value of randomization in experimental design are an outgrowth of three contrary positions on the status of conditionalization, that is, Bayes' theorem, as an inductive postulate. For an illustration of the latter problem I shall point out that techniques for estimating pertinent statistical relations—for example, *Manifest* in DIALOG (a relation that quantitates the association of observable states with a given disease)—are subject to dispute because of the general difficulty of translating the contents of "basic" science into a proper statistical model.

Statistics, as we know it, is a relatively new discipline. Orthodox statistics, those fundamental methods and concepts taught in undergraduate courses, is a twentieth-century product due, primarily, to the work of Jerzy Neyman and Egon S. Pearson. Since about midcentury, however, an old program, now called Bayesianism, has experienced a strong resurgence thanks, mainly, to the efforts of Leonard Savage,

Bruno deFinetti, and Sir Harold Jeffreys. I cannot report in twenty-five words or less the differences between orthodox and Bayesian statistics, but I can discuss one of the important consequences of what I see is the major point of dissension. That consequence is a debate over the value of randomization in experimental design.

A basic result in the mathematical theory of probability is this simplified version of Bayes' theorem:

$$p(A/B) \propto p(B/A) \cdot p(A), \tag{1}$$

the probability of event A, given event B, is proportional to the probability of event B, given event A, multiplied by the (initial) probability of event A. As a theorem of mathematical probability, no one disputes the validity of this statement. But, as Prof. Kyburg correctly reminds us, the problem for inductive logic is to find an acceptable interpretation of formal probability theory. Here, opinions differ about the role Bayes' theorem plays, or ought to play.

Bayesians argue that it specifies an agent's commitments to changes in degrees of belief stemming from a growth in knowledge. For example, if we rewrite the above formula (1) as:

$$p(Disease_i/Manifestation_j) \propto$$

$$p(Manifestation_j/Disease_i) \cdot p(Disease_i), \tag{2}$$

then we discover that the *Evoking* strength of symptom$_j$ for disease$_i$ is proportional to the product of its *Manifest* and the initial plausibility of disease$_i$. Alternatively, we can use Bayes' theorem to guide changes in the *Evoking* strength as more comprehensive sets of manifestations are accumulated. That is, the initial plausibility of disease$_i$ may be understood to be the *Evoking* strength for the disease before adding manifestation$_j$ to the list of observed manifestations, if manifestations of a given disease are probabilistically independent events.

Orthodox statisticians loathe this interpretation of Bayes' theorem, arguing that initial probability is an ill-defined concept: in some cases we fail to know enough to specify an initial probability; in other cases the notion of an initial probability is just inappropriate, a category mistake some would say. Bayesian statisticians are, in principle, never at a loss for precise probabilities, so the orthodox criticisms are easily deflected. If we see the orthodox position uniformly rejecting and the Bayesian position unqualifiedly affirming the validity of Bayes' theorem as an inductive postulate governing changes in rational beliefs, then Prof. Kyburg's original program, epistemological probability, is a compromise. Conditionalization, that is, Bayes' theorem interpreted so as to guide changes in probability with increases in knowledge, is *not* valid epistemologically—but, conditionalization is respected when, by epistemological standards, we have enough precise statistical information for its application, and that is not a rare circumstance.

Among statisticians, probably the most influential figure of the past hundred years is R. A. Fisher. Not wholly affiliated with either the orthodox or the Bayesian program, he is solely responsible for a large number of inductive concepts that have been freely borrowed by one or the other of the two dominant schools. For instance, randomization in experimental design, about which I will have something to say in a few minutes, is one of Fisher's contributions. It is my judgment that Prof. Kyburg's epistemological probability, more than any other theory, serves to reconstruct and ground Fisherian statistics. My immediate goal is to sketch for you how these three positions on conditionalization, that is, the Bayesian, epistemological, and orthodox theories, lead to three different verdicts on randomization.

It is easiest to start by separating Bayesians from the other two groups. Suppose that, as Bayesians, we obtain some compound data that may be decomposed into two parts: d_1 and d_2. The evidence, d_1 & d_2, is possibly relevant to the hypothesis of interest h, and we desire to know the quantitative change in our probability assignment to h as a result of learning these data. Bayes' theorem tells us:

$$p(h/d_1 \ \& \ d_2) \propto p(d_1 \ \& \ d_2/h) \cdot p(h). \tag{3}$$

Suppose, however, that one datum, d_1, probabilistically does not depend upon the hypothesis h. For example, we may be concerned with the bias of a strange coin and have, as new evidence, the tabulation of 100 flips. These data can be summarized concisely by the pair of numbers: d_1, the number of flips ($= 100$); and d_2, the proportion of these 100 flips that land heads up. But we agree that the single datum that the coin was flipped 100 times is probabilistically independent of the hypothesis of the bias of the coin, given the experimental design to stop after 100 flips. That is,

$$p(d_1/h) = p(d_1). \tag{4}$$

As a second example, we may be searching for cases of a novel disease in order to estimate the *Manifest* relations of several of its symptoms, that is, how often does manifestation$_j$ associate with the new disease. If the study turns up exactly 543 histories of the disease, this fact alone is probabilistically independent of the *Manifest* relations.

Formally, define data d, such as these, to be *ancillary* for the hypothesis h whenever d is probabilistically independent of h:

$$p(d/h) = p(d). \tag{5}$$

It is now a simple result that, assuming conditionalization, ancillary data are by themselves absolutely irrelevant to the hypothesis in question.

Proof: Let d be ancillary for h. By Bayes' theorem $p(h/d) \propto p(d/h)$ $p(h)$. But since d is ancillary for h, $p(d/h)$ is a constant (independent of h), $p(d)$, which may be absorbed into the constant of proportionality, leading to:

$$p(h/d) = p(h). \tag{6}$$

In other words, d is irrelevant to h.

What is the significance of this analysis to the debate over randomization? Suppose we consider the report of an experiment designed to test the treatment effects of some procedure. Split the experimental data in two parts: Part one, d_1, reports merely which individual subjects in the experiment fall into the control group and which fall into the treatment group. The other part, d_2, reports the quantitative effects of the treatment versus the controls. Now, if the experiment is rigorously randomized, the division between the treatment and control groups is determined by the randomizer, which, by definition, yields a division that is probabilistically independent of the treatment effects. Hence, to use the randomizer to divide the sample subjects into test and control groups is to make that division ancillary to the test of the treatment effects. That is, by Bayesian standards, the randomization is totally irrelevant once the actual division is effected and made part of the evidence:

$$p(h/d_1 \ \& \ d_2) \propto p(d_1 \ \& \ d_2/h) \cdot p(h) \propto p(d_2/d_1 \ \& \ h) \cdot p(h). \tag{7}$$

Professor Kyburg has summarized this conclusion by noting that the traditional frequency arguments for randomization make sense on a pretrial basis, before we learn the actual treatment/control division of the sample—but those very arguments *may* be valueless (say, as safeguards against bias) on a posttrial analysis, after the sample is divided. Of course Prof. Kyburg is anxious to point out the errors in orthodox statistical methods as a means of highlighting the differences between his original epistemological probability theory and Neyman/Pearson statistics. I remind you, however, that epistemological probability is a position midway between the orthodox and Bayesian inference concerning the role assigned to Bayes' theorem, and thus there are cases where conditionalization is *not* epistemologically valid. It is in those cases that classical randomization is validated on a posttrial interpretation by Prof. Kyburg's theory.

Prof. Kyburg has argued that, epistemologically, randomization is neither necessary nor sufficient for sound inductive inference. He means by that heretical-sounding remark that in some cases it is not necessary and in some cases it is not sufficient. Which cases are these? We have seen that randomization is suspect when conditionalization (or as much of that principle as is required to derive the foregoing result on ancillary information) is sanctioned. Orthodox statistics rejects conditionalization outright when "priors" are denied, and randomization is fully licensed. Bayesian theory takes conditionalization as axiomatic; hence randomization is valueless once the data are reported in their entirety. Epistemological probability denies conditionalization the rank of an inductive postulate, but tolerates it when sufficiently precise frequency information is available, and paralleling this is a tempered stand on randomization. Hence, I conclude that the dispute over the merits of randomization represents a three-sided dialogue stemming from competing attitudes toward a single inductive principle: conditionalization.

I would like now to shift our attention to the second kind of problem I described at the outset: problems that persist for all inductive programs. In his presentation Dr. Donald Seldin has reminded us of the importance of "basic" science for clinical practice. I hope to show that this observation is relevant to my second category of inductive problems.

Let us consider, as an example, the need in DIALOG for estimates of various statistical relations. The program is powerless without quantitative estimates of, say, the *Manifest* relations, and these estimates are based on known frequencies available ahead of time. Each of the statistical theories we have been discussing has its own procedures for solving such simple estimation problems as those posed by DIALOG.

Without going into detail it is fair to say that common to all is the conclusion that *more is better;* that is, more data make for better estimates.

Bayesians appeal to notions of stable estimation: the interpersonal convergence of estimates with increasing evidence. It is the standard desideratum of a good estimation procedure. Orthodox statisticians make use of the asymptotic performance (asymptotic with increasing sample size) to gauge the merits of different estimators. After all, what is intuitively wrong with the requirement that estimates should improve with increases in the empirical content of the evidential input used for calculating the estimates?

The challenge I want to raise can be illustrated by a recent, perplexing result (hinted at in B. Efron and C. Morris, "Stein's Paradox in Statistics," *Scientific American,* May 1977, 119–128). When estimating a large number of statistical relations—for example, all the *Manifest* values—improvements in the individual estimates of separate *Manifest* relations can be had by considering all the *Manifest* values at once. Thus, the estimate of $M(M_1,D_1)$ is affected by the observed frequencies for $M(M_1,D_2)$, or by the frequencies for $M(M_2,D_3)$, even when M_1 is not a manifestation of disease D_3!

Clearly the guide that more is better gets out of hand when this procedure makes statistical sense. I suggest that the problem here – one to be on guard against, no matter which inductive logic is your favorite—is the simple point that the statistical populations used to model the medical phenomena (in DIALOG) are handy idealizations that fail to capture all the important content of the basic medical science available for explanation of those phenomena. What I am trying to say is that the rule of thumb should read: more of the same sort of data makes for better estimates. The disturbing point is that, from the standpoint of the basic science, what count as statistically similar data are really distinct.

Statistical inference is a wonderful tool for analyzing numerical relations within what loosely is called a *population.* But one need not have much background knowledge in order to specify a population and to digest numbers pertaining to it in a statistically meaningful way. The danger I allude to arises when we do have a rich stock of scientific background that may not be adequately reflected in the simplified statistical model used. I do not know of a formal mechanism adequate for evaluating the "fit" between a basic science and its statistical model. Nonetheless, I hope I have alerted the users of DIALOG to one of the dangers that attends the application of extra sensitive statistical techniques when those techniques outrun the accuracy in the statistical modeling of the available basic science.

PART TWO

INTERNIST and CADUCEUS

8

The Process of Clinical Diagnosis and Its Adaptation to the Computer*

Jack D. Myers

Some seven years ago, upon a change of career, the author was fortunate to team up with Dr. Harry Pople and begin to devise a diagnostic program for internal medicine using the techniques of "artificial intelligence." This resulted in much more introspection in regard to my own diagnostic processes, and my behavior as a physician changed somewhat as a result of that introspection. This is reflected in the following comments about the process of clinical diagnosis. The process is examined through my own eyes and experience, but let me assure the reader that I am a fairly orthodox internist, and the observations should apply quite generally. Second, I shall turn to a discussion of how the process of clinical diagnosis has been applied to the INTERNIST-I schema, although many details of that will be left for Dr. Pople's later presentation. Third, there will be an illustration of an actual computer case analysis.

There are several classical stages to the process of clinical diagnosis. The first of these, of course, is information gathering. Some call it cue acquisition, which we gain from taking a history from the patient, doing the physical examination, and performing various varieties of laboratory investigation. In general the physician tries to use the simpler, cheaper, and less dangerous approaches first, and he will resort

*Supported by Research Grant 5 R24 RR01101 from the Division of Research Resources, National Institutes of Health.

to others only when there is a significant potential gain diagnostically and in terms of patient management particularly. One of the obvious problems with this information gathering is the reliability of the information. Errors are made both of commission and of omission, but it should be emphasized that general experience indicates that the errors in information gathering usually are not nearly of the magnitude or seriousness as are the errors in interpretation of the information that is gathered, or as are the errors of hypothesis formation from the information. Nevertheless, there is in the information on any given patient a certain degree of unreliability, and one of the decisions the physician must make is what part of this information to disregard in his analytical reasoning. Some physicians tend to be very comprehensive in their information gathering—some to the point where the comprehensiveness clutters the mind with irrelevant information and actually hampers the diagnostic process (information overload). Accordingly, most physicians tend to gather information in a more limited and directed fashion. And generally, the better the diagnostician, in my experience, the more this factor applies. In fact, the good diagnostician, in the early stages of collection of information, promptly forms certain hypotheses on the basis of the incomplete information, and the information gathering from then on is greatly influenced by those early hypotheses. They may be significantly modified, of course, as the process proceeds. One important factor, then, in the process of clinical diagnosis is that the information gathering is greatly influenced by the ideas the diagnostician has regarding the problem before him.

Once the information has been gathered, several hypotheses have already been generated in regard to the information—the initial differential diagnosis, if you will. One of the ways by which the clinician does this is to reflect on the mass of information he has gathered and to identify certain cardinal features in this information. Obviously, the most telling cardinal feature would be one that is exclusive or pathognomonic for a given disease, but these are not common. Nevertheless, there are other cardinal features that point strongly but not exclusively to a given diagnosis. When cardinal features are lacking, and often they are, then the diagnostician groups various pieces of the information into clusters of items and weighs these mentally as supporting or denying the various hypotheses that have been generated. Some physicians in this respect deal only with positive information, and they will derive a cluster or a list of positive items that points to disease A. A more refined physician will subtract from that positive list the negative items, those that do not fit with the given hypothesis; and this, I believe, is a superior approach. One of the traps at this particular level, however, is that some of the pieces of information may not be interpreted at all; they may be very important but are overlooked either temporarily or sometimes on a more lasting basis. Other pieces may be misinterpreted, but it should be reemphasized that considerable error is produced in the process by the overlooking or lack of interpretation of certain pieces of information.

The working memory of the clinician usually can deal with up to about five diagnostic hypotheses at any one time. Only the more brilliant are able to exceed this number. Studies have shown that seven is probably about the maximal number that an individual can deal with in his working memory at any one time. He may shift gears, of course, as he moves from one set of hypotheses to another, but he won't necessarily be considering fourteen processes at the same time. If the number he is considering is on the larger end of the seven, the clinician often seeks information, extant or additional, by which to delete certain hypotheses from the list, to rule out certain of the hypotheses. When he gets down to two or three hypotheses, he looks for information that will tend to separate these hypotheses—to support one or deny another. When he is down to one hypothesis, or he may be dealing with only one hypothesis from the beginning for that matter, he looks for confirmatory evidence to support that hypothesis, and finding it he makes a diagnosis. If he does not confirm the hypothesis, he reverts to another hypothesis or to a list of them.

In this process, there generally are several principles that the diagnostician follows. First, he likes to believe that he is reasoning with the information base regarding a patient on a pathophysiological basis. In other words, he is dealing with the evidence at a level of basic understanding through physiology or pathology. It turns out, however, that in the majority of instances the clinician does not do this. He does this overtly in about one-third of the diagnostic problems with which he deals. In the others, perhaps subconsciously he deals with the pathophysiological explanation for the evidence, but he tends to jump over that consideration and comes to diagnostic conclusions without consciously taking account of pathophysiology. It is of interest that, when Dr. Pople and I first began to work with INTERNIST-I, we adopted the attitude that all evidence should be explained in pathophysiological terms. But after about a year it became evident that that was an extremely costly and often wasteful procedure. Our program still has a strong element of pathophysiology as its base, but, as you will see, it does not have to consider all the elements of evidence in making a step from A to B. It skips over A' and A". In the most difficult problems, however, the expert clinician usually does resort to pathophysiological reasoning and explanation.

A second principle is that, by and large, one likes to proceed in orderly fashion from a general consideration to a specific consideration. Let me explain what I mean by an example. One can conclude on evidence that the patient has some form of heart failure, but what kind is not clear. It is proper then to ask the question, "Does the heart failure involve the heart valves or the heart muscle or the pericardial sac?" If one decides that it is a valvular problem, one can focus on the particular valve and the particular disorder. This process does not need to be followed all the time, but it is a very good approach in a difficult diagnostic setting.

A third principle is what I call Stead's rule because I learned it from Dr. Eugene Stead, my mentor at Harvard, Emory, and Duke. Stead's rule is that common diseases are common. And so one tends to give some degree of preference to a disease that has a high frequency in the population rather than to some rare disorder. One has to be cautious about this, however, because in dealing with the statistics regarding a single patient, we always have that factor of $n-1$ in the denominator. When n, the number of patients under consideration, is 1, $n-1$ equals 0, and you cannot divide by zero. So error can be introduced into the diagnostic process by too much emphasis on commonality.

Lastly, one has the factor of the practical considerations of the situation. How seriously ill does the patient seem to be? Is there an emergency here? Does the problem one is dealing with involve some satisfactory treatment? Dr. Samuel Levine, one of my teachers at Harvard many years ago, always followed this principle. He would say, "I do not care whether I make a diagnosis of multiple sclerosis; there is little I can do about it anyway. I want to make sure that this patient does not have a tumor of the spinal cord which we can remove surgically and cure the patient." Most of us follow this principle of the pragmatic aspects of the problem to some degree or other.

Now let me turn to how some of these points are translated into INTERNIST-I. INTERNIST-I is currently confined to internal medicine, and it includes about 750 diagnostic nodes, of which some 500 are terminal-disease nodes (May 1984). First, we have to classify these many disorders. We start with a very broad category like liver disease and make subdivisions expressed in fairly broad terms, such as hepatic parenchymal disease, cholestasis, hepatic vascular disease, hereditary hyperbilirubinemia, and so on. Then, for example, cholestasis is divided into two large categories, obstruction of large ducts and obstruction of small ducts within the liver. Next the large-duct obstruction is finally divided into specific disease categories, carcinoma of the bile duct, carcinoma of the head of the pancreas, sclerosing cholangitis, choledocholithiasis, stricture of the bile duct, and so on. This classification has the potential of allowing one to progress from the general to the specific in the diagnostic process.

Each individual disease is profiled. Table 1 is a partial list, a very partial list, of the findings of choledocholithiasis, one or more gall stones in the common bile duct. The list for this disease is currently sixty-three manifestations long. There are two numbers after each manifestation. The first number is termed the evoking strength, and it asks the question, "If the patient has that manifestation of disease, how likely is this specific diagnosis?" on a scale of 1 to 5, with 5 being maximal. There are some 0's as first numbers. That means that the manifestation, such as weight loss—the second item—is so spread among diseases that it has little specificity in diagnosis. So no evoking strength is assigned. Arranging our medical information in these six

TABLE 1

SELECTED MANIFESTATIONS UNDER CHOLEDOCHOLITHIASIS

Jaundice intermittent HX	2	3
Weight loss gtr than 10 percent	0	1
Abdomen pain colicky	2	3
Vomiting recent	0	3
Jaundice	2	3
Liver enlarged moderate	2	3
SGOT 120 to 400	1	1
Bile duct cholangiography common duct and/or intrahepatic duct (S) dilated	3	3
Bile duct cholangiography common duct round filling defect (S)	4	4
Liver biopsy bile plugging	2	4

categories is not at all difficult. If, however, one tries to go much higher in refining it, one would run into a limitation of information. It is important to emphasize that the incidence of diseases used for estimation of evoking strengths is that for the temperate zones of North America and Europe. The medical knowledge base would require significant revision if it were to be used in the tropics, for example, where the distribution of diseases is quite different.

The second numbers are termed the frequency numbers, and they ask the question, "If the disease is present, how likely is the manifestation?" Again the numbers range from 1 to 5, 1 being rare or unusual, 2 meaning a significant minority, 3 about half, 4 a significant majority and 5 essentially all. The next to the last item in Table 1, where cholangiography shows round filling defects, which are usually stones, has a first number of 4, which indicates that a majority of patients with this X-ray finding will have choledocholithiasis. There are some errors in the procedure due to gas bubbles, and thus that number is not a 5. The second number of 4 indicates that a majority of patients who have choledocholithiasis, if examined for these defects, will demonstrate them. These numbers are used heavily by the computer diagnostic system.

The data can be rearranged by manifestation rather than by disease. Table 2 illustrates those specific diseases thus far profiled that produce massive enlargement of the spleen. The first and second numbers are the same as detailed above. One can readily observe that, among these diseases, chronic myelocytic leukemia is the most common cause of massive splenomegaly but that myeloid metaplasia produces the splenomegaly more frequently. Both the orientation of this information by disease and its orientation by manifestation are useful ways of storing and retrieving medical information and have distinct educational application.

There is a third important number that is assigned. This is termed the importance or "import" and again ranges from 1 to 5, 5 being maximal. The number answers a global question: "How important in general is this manifestation of disease in diagnosis, must it be explained, or how readily can it be disregarded?" Obviously, any manifestation that does not fit into a diagnosis and has a low importance can be disregarded, and the computer system can do so.

Manifestations are classified in order to deal with the problem, which I mentioned earlier, of not doing expensive, dangerous procedures first and before simpler measures are reasonably exhausted.

TABLE 2

DISEASES EVOKED BY A MANIFESTATION SPLENOMEGALY MASSIVE

Amyloidosis systemic	1	1
Sarcoidosis chronic systemic	1	1
Histoplasmosis disseminated	1	1
Leukemia hairy cell	1	3
Lymphosarcoma	2	1
Hodgkins disease systemic	1	1
Leukemia chronic lymphocytic	1	1
Leukemia acute lymphoblastic	1	1
Waldenstroms Macroglobulinemia	1	1
Leukemia chronic myelocytic in blastic crisis	2	2
Leukemia chronic myelocytic	3	2
Myeloid metaplasia	2	3
Paroxysmal nocturnal hemoglobinuria	1	1
Presinusoidal portal hypertension	1	1
Sinusoidal or postsinusoidal portal hypertension	1	1

Manifestations are classified as historical items, symptoms, physical signs, LAB 0 (routine laboratory procedures which essentially every hospitalized patient undergoes), LAB 1 (laboratory procedures that are not routine but also not expensive or invasive) and LAB 2 (laboratory procedures that are very expensive, very uncomfortable, and/or invasive). LAB 2 procedures are invoked by the computer system only when necessary for diagnosis.

Last, there are a number of other "properties" that are assigned to the various manifestations of disease, such as prerequisites. For example, testicular tenderness would be looked for only in a male and not in a female, and so forth. There are many implications that the program has to know; if A is true, B is also true and C is not true. For example, if the system knows that a patient has a high serum cholesterol, it does not inquire about or consider a low serum cholesterol.

The system, having been provided information about a patient in the form of manifestations of disease, will formulate, just as in real life, various models or hypotheses regarding diagnosis. There are four lists of manifestations for each model evoked. List A includes manifestations present in the patient and explained by the disease. This list supports that hypothesis; the evoking strengths, the first numbers indicating how strongly each positive manifestation makes one consider a disease hypothesis among all others, are used here to give mathematical value to List A. List B contains manifestations present in the patient but not explained by the disease. These may be red herrings or they may be explained by some second disease that the patient has; here the import numbers are used to quantitate B. List C consists of manifestations expected in the disease but not found present in the patient. The list counts against the disease; here the second numbers, the frequency of the manifestation given the disease, are the values utilized. And last, List D is composed of manifestations expected in the disease but not known about one way or another; that allows the system to go into an interrogative mode, and depending on the answers, one or more of lists A, B, and C are modified. Thus each hypothesis or disease model has a net mathematical value and a rank relative to other diseases evoked.

Most importantly, the evoked models are then partitioned in INTERNIST-I, partitioned so that the system is comparing apples with apples and oranges with oranges. For example, one does not want to compare a stone in the common bile duct with congestive heart failure. The patient, if there is evidence for both of those, will have two disorders. The partitioning system in oversimplification depends on homology: where two or more disease models are homologous, they are competitors; but if they are not, they are regarded as possibly both being present, that is, as complementary.

The system next selects a mode of analysis for the leading partition. If there are many evoked hypotheses and none of them predominate, it goes into a *Rule-out* mode and for each evoked disease will ask questions that have a high frequency number in order to rule a given hypothesis either in or out. When the list within the leading partition is reduced to a few strong possibilities, a *Discriminate* mode is evoked. Here questions are asked that will either support one disease and at the same time downgrade another or vice versa. In this mode both numbers, the evoking strengths and the frequency numbers, are utilized. Last, when one leading contender emerges (or this may occur initially as the models are set up, provided one is strong enough), a *Pursue* mode comes into force to try to confirm that diagnosis. The evoking strengths are the numbers that are used to select questions.

Once the first diagnosis is concluded, the manifestations explained by that disease are eliminated, and the whole process recycles in order to use the remaining, unexplained manifestations and to make additional diagnoses whenever the evidence is adequate. But before it recycles, bonus values called "links" are awarded to any other disease related to the disease already concluded. Such "links" are very important in the diagnostic process because of the advisability of diagnosing related rather than independent diseases whenever the evidence justifies.

Dr. Pople and I, after our initial exploration, came to the conclusion that a diagnostic system in internal medicine had to meet at least five characteristics: (1) the ability to make multiple diagnoses related or independent, (2) the *ad hoc* construction of the diagnostic complex (because no two patients are ever exactly alike, each diagnostic problem is to a greater or lesser degree unique), (3) indifference to the order of presentation of information (because information usually does not come to the physician in an orderly fashion), (4) progression from the general to the specific, which is often but not always advisable, and (5) ability to disregard irrelevancies. The current INTERNIST-I program meets all of these qualifications except for number four.

A case analysis is the best method to illustrate the operation of INTERNIST-I. The example chosen is a case from the Massachusetts General Hospital (Scully 1978, 466). The diagnostic problem is summarized so that the reader can observe how the computer program deals with it. The case is that of a young woman who turns out to have progressive systemic sclerosis (PSS) involving the kidneys. Incidentally, *scleroderma* is a commonly used synonym for *progressive systemic sclerosis*. The reason this case was difficult and was published is that the patient clinically did not show any good or convincing evidence of the disease except within the kidneys. Most of the time PSS is a quite widespread systemic disorder, but in this patient the process was essentially confined to the kidneys. In fact, the only other place the disease was identified was in the skin of the wrist, when a surgeon did a cutdown in order to inaugurate a renal dialysis procedure on the patient and noticed that the tissue was tough. He reported this to the internist, and when the surgeon had to reorganize the shunt, he took a biopsy and found the typical fibrosis of scleroderma. The correct diagnosis was made at the Massachusetts General Hospital only by a kidney biopsy. The reader should observe the parallelism between the human experience and the machine performance. Initially, the information from the patient just as it appears in the protocol is entered into the computer.

Initial positive manifestations (findings present in the patient):

```
SEX FEMALE
AGE 26 TO 55
LEG (S) EDEMA BILATERAL SLIGHT OR MODERATE
DYSPNEA EXERTIONAL
BACK PAIN SEVERE
URINE DARK HX
PROTEINURIA
PENICILLIN OR SEMI SYNTHETIC PENICILLIN ADMINISTRATION
    RECENT HX
CONTRACEPTIVE ORAL ADMINISTRATION RECENT HX
DIURETIC ADMINISTRATION RECENT HX
UREA NITROGEN BLOOD 30 TO 59
UREA NITROGEN BLOOD 60 TO 100
URINE OUTPUT LESS THAN 400 ML PER DAY
HEART MURMUR HX
HAND (S) XRAY CONGENITAL SKELETAL DEFECT (S)
PRESSURE ARTERIAL DIASTOLIC GTR THAN 125
ORTHOPNEA
CHEST PERCUSSION DULL LOCALIZED
RALES LOCALIZED
HEART MURMUR SYSTOLIC SECOND LEFT INTERSPACE
HEART SOUND (S) S2 SPLITTING WIDE AND FIXED
HEART SOUND (S) S3 LEFT VENTRICULAR GALLOP
ABDOMEN TENDERNESS RIGHT LOWER QUADRANT
ABDOMEN TENDERNESS LEFT UPPER QUADRANT
BACK TENDERNESS COSTOVERTEBRAL ANGLE (S)
PULSE (S) RADIAL DECREASED
URINE SEDIMENT RBC
URINE SEDIMENT WBC
URINE SEDIMENT BROAD CAST (S)
URINE SEDIMENT COARSE GRANULAR CAST (S)
URINE SEDIMENT RENAL TUBULAR CELL CAST (S)
HEMATOCRIT BLOOD LESS THAN 35
WBC 4,000 TO 13,900 PERCENT NEUTROPHIL (S) INCREASED
UREA NITROGEN BLOOD GTR THAN 100
CREATININE BLOOD INCREASED
PHOSPHATE BLOOD INCREASED
URIC ACID BLOOD INCREASED
ELECTROPHORESIS SERUM ALBUMIN DECREASED
BICARBONATE BLOOD LESS THAN 20
LDH BLOOD INCREASED
EKG HEART BLOCK FIRST DEGREE
EKG T WAVE (S) INVERTED
HEART XRAY LEFT VENTRICLE ENLARGED
CHEST XRAY VASCULAR MARKING (S) INCREASED DIFFUSE
CHEST XRAY PLEURAL EFFUSION (S)
```

```
HEART XRAY LEFT ATRIUM ENLARGED MODERATE
HEART XRAY MAIN PULMONARY ARTERY ENLARGED
HEART ECHOCARDIOGRAPHY RIGHT VENTRICLE END-DIASTOLIC
    INTERNAL DIAMETER GTR THAN 2.3 CM
HEART ECHOCARDIOGRAPHY VENTRICULAR SEPTUM PARADOXIC
    SYSTOLIC MOTION
HEART ECHOCARDIOGRAPHY LEFT ATRIUM INTERNAL DIAMETER
    4 TO 6 CM
HEART ECHOCARDIOGRAPHY LEFT VENTRICLE END-DIASTOLIC
    INTERNAL DIAMETER GTR THAN 5.6 CM
BLEEDING TIME INCREASED
FACTOR VIII ANTIHEMOPHILIC INCREASED
RBC RETICULOCYTE (S) GTR THAN 5 PERCENT
HAPTOGLOBIN PLASMA DECREASED
RBC SCHIZOCYTE (S) NUMEROUS
LUNG (S) FORCED VITAL CAPACITY DECREASED
LUNG (S) RESIDUAL VOLUME INCREASED
LUNG (S) FEV1 DECREASED
FIBRINOGEN DEGRADATION PRODUCT (S) BLOOD GTR THAN
    25 MCG PER ML
```

Initial negative findings (Findings not present in the patient):

```
BACK PAIN RADIATING TO POSTERIOR THIGH
PROTEINURIA HX
RIGOR (S)
PHARYNGITIS RECENT HX
IMPETIGO HX
JOINT (S) PAIN MILD TRANSIENT
SKIN RASH MACULOPAPULAR
SCALP ALOPECIA
RAYNAUDS PHENOMENON
DYSPHAGIA SOLID (S)
DYSPHAGIA LIQUID (S)
HYPERTENSION HX
HYPERTENSION FAMILY HX
KIDNEY DISEASE FAMILY HX
DEAFNESS FAMILY HX
HEART DISEASE FAMILY HX
FEVER
TACHYCARDIA
TACHYPNEA
SKIN THICK INDURATED
PRESSURE VENOUS INCREASED ON INSPECTION
LYMPH NODE (S) ENLARGED
LIVER ENLARGED SLIGHT
LIVER ENLARGED MODERATE
SPLENOMEGALY SLIGHT
SPLENOMEGALY MODERATE
PLATELETS 50,000 TO 200,000
PLATELETS LESS THAN 50,000
```

```
PROTHROMBIN TIME INCREASED
ACTIVATED PARTIAL THROMBOPLASTIN TIME INCREASED
GLUCOSE BLOOD 130 TO 300
CALCIUM BLOOD INCREASED
CALCIUM BLOOD DECREASED
BILIRUBIN BLOOD CONJUGATED INCREASED
SGOT 40 TO 119
CPK BLOOD INCREASED
AMYLASE BLOOD INCREASED
ALKALINE PHOSPHATASE BLOOD INCREASED NOT OVER
    2 TIMES NORMAL
ABDOMEN XRAY FLUID PERITONEAL CAVITY DIFFUSE
KIDNEY (S) FLAT FILM SMALL BILATERAL
KIDNEY (S) ULTRASONOGRAPHY SMALL BILATERAL
KIDNEY (S) ULTRASONOGRAPHY PELVIS (ES) DILATED
HEART ECHOCARDIOGRAPHY PERICARDIAL EFFUSION
THROAT CULTURE STREPTOCOCCUS BETA HEMOLYTIC
COOMBS TEST DIRECT POSITIVE
RHEUMATOID FACTOR POSITIVE
ANA POSITIVE
HEPATITIS B SURFACE ANTIGEN
ANTIBODY HEPATITIS B SURFACE ANTIGEN
ANTIBODY STREPTOLYSIN O INCREASED
VISCOSITY SERUM INCREASED
COMPLEMENT C3 SERUM DECREASED
COMPLEMENT C4 SERUM DECREASED
CRYOGLOBULIN (S) BLOOD INCREASED
VITAMIN B12 SERUM LESS THAN 100
FOLATE SERUM LESS THAN 3
LUNG (S) CAPACITY TOTAL INCREASED
CARBON DIOXIDE TENSION BLOOD ARTERIAL INCREASED
GROWTH RETARDATION
```

(It can be readily observed that this is a list of miscellaneous information. All of the reported positive and negative manifestations are entered. Note that among the negatives is Raynaud's phenomenon, which is found frequently in patients with PSS. Also note that the skin was not thick and indurated on physical examination as it is classically in PSS.)

```
DISREGARDING:  BACK PAIN SEVERE, DYSPNEA EXERTIONAL,
ORTHOPNEA, ABDOMEN TENDERNESS RIGHT LOWER QUADRANT,
CHEST PERCUSSION DULL LOCALIZED, HAND (S) XRAY
CONGENITAL SKELETAL DEFECT (S), HEART MURMUR SYSTOLIC
SECOND LEFT INTERSPACE, HEART SOUND (S) S2 SPLITTING
WIDE AND FIXED, HEART SOUND (S) S3 LEFT VENTRICULAR
GALLOP, PULSE (S) RADIAL DECREASED, RALES LOCALIZED,
BICARBONATE BLOOD LESS THAN 20, CHEST XRAY PLEURAL
EFFUSION (S), CHEST XRAY VASCULAR MARKING (S)
INCREASED DIFFUSE, EKG HEART BLOCK FIRST DEGREE,
```

```
HEART XRAY LEFT ATRIUM ENLARGED MODERATE, HEART XRAY
MAIN PULMONARY ARTERY ENLARGED, PHOSPHATE BLOOD
INCREASED, RBC SCHIZOCYTE (S) NUMEROUS, UREA NITROGEN
BLOOD GTR THAN 100, FACTOR VIII ANTIHEMOPHILIC
INCREASED, FIBRINOGEN DEGRADATION PRODUCT (S) BLOOD
GTR THAN 25 MCG PER ML, HAPTOGLOBIN PLASMA DECREASED,
HEART ECHOCARDIOGRAPHY LEFT ATRIUM INTERNAL DIAMETER
4 TO 6 CM, HEART ECHOCARDIOGRAPHY LEFT VENTRICLE END-
DIASTOLIC INTERNAL DIAMETER GTR THAN 5.6 CM, HEART
ECHOCARDIOGRAPHY RIGHT VENTRICLE END-DIASTOLIC
INTERNAL DIAMETER GTR THAN 2.3 CM, HEART ECHOCARDIOG-
RAPHY VENTRICULAR SEPTUM PARADOXIC SYSTOLIC MOTION,
LUNG (S) FEV1 DECREASED, LUNG (S) FORCED VITAL
CAPACITY DECREASED, RBC RETICULOCYTE (S) GTR THAN
5 PERCENT, LUNG (S) RESIDUAL VOLUME INCREASED

CONSIDERING:  AGE 26 TO 55, CONTRACEPTIVE ORAL ADMIN-
ISTRATION RECENT HX, SEX FEMALE, BACK TENDERNESS
COSTOVERTEBRAL ANGLE (S), LEG (S) EDEMA BILATERAL
SLIGHT OR MODERATE, PRESSURE ARTERIAL DIASTOLIC GTR
THAN 125, CREATININE BLOOD INCREASED, HEART XRAY LEFT
VENTRICLE ENLARGED, HEMATOCRIT BLOOD LESS THAN 35,
PROTEINURIA, UREA NITROGEN BLOOD 30 TO 59, UREA
NITROGEN BLOOD 60 TO 100, URIC ACID BLOOD INCREASED,
URINE OUTPUT LESS THAN 400 ML PER DAY, URINE SEDIMENT
BROAD CAST (S), URINE SEDIMENT COARSE GRANULAR CAST
(S), URINE SEDIMENT RBC, URINE SEDIMENT RENAL TUBULAR
CELL CAST (S), URINE SEDIMENT WBC, WBC 4,000 TO
13,900 PERCENT NEUTROPHIL (S) INCREASED, ELECTRO-
PHORESIS SERUM ALBUMIN DECREASED

RULEOUT:  PROGRESSIVE SYSTEMIC SCLEROSIS INVOLVING
KIDNEYS, GLOMERULONEPHRITIS ADVANCED CHRONIC, DIABETIC
NEPHROPATHY, GLOMERULONEPHRITIS ACUTE, RENAL
VASCULITIS
```

(Certain disease models have been evoked with attention first directed toward the kidney involvement. The *Rule-out* mode of analysis tells us that there are at least five contenders and that at this point none is predominantly strong. Strikingly, however, PSS involving the kidneys is in first place. The several forms of glomerulonephritis and diabetic neuropathy are all considerably more common diseases. PSS involving the kidneys explains all of the items on the "Considering" list, which applies only to the first diagnosis listed and not necessarily and completely to the competitors. The "Disregarding" list is composed of items that are not explained by PSS involving the kidneys; most of these manifestations will be dealt with later in the analysis.

The system now enters an interrogative phase seeking further information in order to try to eliminate some of the contenders and to reduce the list to more definitive proportions. The absence of a history of diabetes is evidence against diabetic nephropathy. The abrupt onset of hypertension supports PSS but also acute glomerulonephritis and renal vasculitis; the frequency number, however, is highest for PSS. The system inquires about weight loss, but the system is instructed to "yield" to the operator because the patient had sustained a recent weight gain. The weight increase proves not to be very critical information in this setting.)

```
DIABETES MELLITUS HX?
NO

PLEASE ENTER FINDINGS OF BLOOD PRESSURE
*GO
```

(The operator can enter any data he has on this subject. No additional information being proffered, the command "GO" turns the initiative back to the computer.)

```
HYPERTENSION ABRUPT ONSET?
YES

PLEASE ENTER FINDINGS OF APPETITE/WEIGHT
*GO

WEIGHT LOSS GTR THAN 10 PERCENT?
YIELD

*WEIGHT INCREASE RECENT HX

*GO

DISREGARDING:  WEIGHT INCREASE RECENT HX, BACK PAIN
SEVERE, DYSPNEA EXERTIONAL, ORTHOPNEA, ABDOMEN TENDER-
NESS RIGHT LOWER QUADRANT, CHEST PERCUSSION DULL
LOCALIZED, HAND (S) XRAY CONGENITAL SKELETAL DEFECT
(S), HEART MURMUR SYSTOLIC SECOND LEFT INTERSPACE,
HEART SOUND (S) S2 SPLITTING WIDE AND FIXED, HEART
SOUND (S) S3 LEFT VENTRICULAR GALLOP, PULSE (S) RADIAL
DECREASED, RALES LOCALIZED, BICARBONATE BLOOD LESS
THAN 20, CHEST XRAY PLEURAL EFFUSION (S), CHEST XRAY
VASCULAR MARKING (S) INCREASED DIFFUSE, EKG HEART
BLOCK FIRST DEGREE, HEART XRAY LEFT ATRIUM ENLARGED
MODERATE, HEART XRAY MAIN PULMONARY ARTERY ENLARGED,
PHOSPHATE BLOOD INCREASED, RBC SCHIZOCYTE (S) NUMER-
OUS, UREA NITROGEN BLOOD GTR THAN 100, FACTOR VIII
ANTIHEMOPHILIC INCREASED, FIBRINOGEN DEGRADATION
```

```
PRODUCT (S) BLOOD GTR THAN 25 MCG PER ML, HAPTOGLOBIN
PLASMA DECREASED, HEART ECHOCARDIOGRAPHY LEFT ATRIUM
INTERNAL DIAMETER 4 TO 6 CM, HEART ECHOCARDIOGRAPHY
LEFT VENTRICLE END-DIASTOLIC INTERNAL DIAMETER GTR
THAN 5.6 CM, HEART ECHOCARDIOGRAPHY RIGHT VENTRICLE
END-DIASTOLIC INTERNAL DIAMETER GTR THAN 2.3 CM, HEART
ECHOCARDIOGRAPHY VENTRICULAR SEPTUM PARADOXIC SYSTOLIC
MOTION, LUNG (S) FEV1 DECREASED, LUNG (S) FORCED VITAL
CAPACITY DECREASED, RBC RETICULOCYTE (S) GTR THAN
5 PERCENT, LUNG (S) RESIDUAL VOLUME INCREASED

CONSIDERING:   AGE 26 TO 55, CONTRACEPTIVE ORAL ADMIN-
ISTRATION RECENT HX, HYPERTENSION ABRUPT ONSET, SEX
FEMALE, BACK TENDERNESS COSTOVERTEBRAL ANGLE (S),
LEG (S), EDEMA BILATERAL SLIGHT OR MODERATE, PRESSURE
ARTERIAL DIASTOLIC GTR THAN 125, CREATININE BLOOD
INCREASED, HEART XRAY LEFT VENTRICLE ENLARGED,
HEMATOCRIT BLOOD LESS THAN 35, PROTEINURIA, UREA
NITROGEN BLOOD 30 TO 59, UREA NITROGEN BLOOD 60 TO
100, URIC ACID BLOOD INCREASED, URINE OUTPUT LESS THAN
400 ML PER DAY, URINE SEDIMENT BROAD CAST (S), URINE
SEDIMENT COARSE GRANULAR CAST (S), URINE SEDIMENT RBC,
URINE SEDIMENT RENAL TUBULAR CELL CAST (S), URINE
SEDIMENT WBC, WBC 4,000 TO 13,900 PERCENT NEUTROPHIL
(S) INCREASED, ELECTROPHORESIS SERUM ALBUMIN DECREASED

DISCRIMINATE:   PROGRESSIVE SYSTEMIC SCLEROSIS INVOLV-
ING KIDNEYS, GLOMERULONEPHRITIS ADVANCED CHRONIC
```

(The system is now in the *Discriminate* mode, meaning that two leading contenders have evolved from analysis of the information available at this time. Five questions are asked, the answers to which to some degree favor one or the other of the two leading contenders. For example, a decreased blood potassium is occasionally found in PSS but not in chronic glomerulonephritis.)

```
PLEASE ENTER FINDINGS OF URINALYSIS ROUTINE AND
   MICROSCOPIC
*GO

URINE HEMATURIA GROSS WITH MICROSCOPIC CONFIRMATION?
NO

PLEASE ENTER FINDINGS OF ELECTROLYTE (S) SERUM
*GO

POTASSIUM BLOOD DECREASED?
NO
```

```
URINE SPECIFIC GRAVITY 1:008 TO 1:014?
N/A
```

(N/A means not available—no information about this specific item.)

```
PLEASE ENTER FINDINGS OF EYE (S) EXTERNAL EXAM
*GO

EYE (S) EDEMA PERIORBITAL?
NO

GLYCOSURIA?
NO

DISREGARDING:  WEIGHT INCREASE RECENT HX, BACK PAIN
SEVERE, DYSPNEA EXERTIONAL, ORTHOPNEA, ABDOMEN TENDER-
NESS RIGHT LOWER QUADRANT, CHEST PERCUSSION DULL
LOCALIZED, HAND (S) XRAY CONGENITAL SKELETAL DEFECT
(S), HEART MURMUR SYSTOLIC SECOND LEFT INTERSPACE,
HEART SOUND (S) S2 SPLITTING WIDE AND FIXED, HEART
SOUND (S) S3 LEFT VENTRICULAR GALLOP, PULSE (S) RADIAL
DECREASED, RALES LOCALIZED, BICARBONATE BLOOD LESS
THAN 20, CHEST XRAY PLEURAL EFFUSION (S), CHEST XRAY
VASCULAR MARKING (S) INCREASED DIFFUSE, EKG HEART
BLOCK FIRST DEGREE, HEART XRAY LEFT ATRIUM ENLARGED
MODERATE, HEART XRAY MAIN PULMONARY ARTERY ENLARGED,
PHOSPHATE BLOOD INCREASED, RBC SCHIZOCYTE (S) NUMER-
OUS, UREA NITROGEN BLOOD GTR THAN 100, FACTOR VIII
ANTIHEMOPHILIC INCREASED, FIBRINOGEN DEGRADATION
PRODUCT (S) BLOOD GTR THAN 25 MCG PER ML, HAPTOGLOBIN
PLASMA DECREASED, HEART ECHOCARDIOGRAPHY LEFT ATRIUM
INTERNAL DIAMETER 4 TO 6 CM, HEART ECHOCARDIOGRAPHY
LEFT VENTRICLE END-DIASTOLIC INTERNAL DIAMETER GTR
THAN 5.6 CM, HEART ECHOCARDIOGRAPHY RIGHT VENTRICLE
END-DIASTOLIC INTERNAL DIAMETER GTR THAN 2.3 CM, HEART
ECHOCARDIOGRAPHY VENTRICULAR SEPTUM PARADOXIC SYSTOLIC
MOTION, LUNG (S) FEV1 DECREASED, LUNG (S) FORCED VITAL
CAPACITY DECREASED, RBC RETICULOCYTE (S) GTR THAN
5 PERCENT, LUNG (S) RESIDUAL VOLUME INCREASED

CONSIDERING:  AGE 26 TO 55, CONTRACEPTIVE ORAL ADMIN-
ISTRATION RECENT HX, HYPERTENSION ABRUPT ONSET, SEX
FEMALE, BACK TENDERNESS COSTOVERTEBRAL ANGLE (S),
LEG (S) EDEMA BILATERAL SLIGHT OR MODERATE, PRESSURE
ARTERIAL DIASTOLIC GTR THAN 125, CREATININE BLOOD
INCREASED, HEART XRAY LEFT VENTRICLE ENLARGED,
HEMATOCRIT BLOOD LESS THAN 35, PROTEINURIA, UREA
NITROGEN BLOOD 30 TO 59, UREA NITROGEN BLOOD 60 TO
100, URIC ACID BLOOD INCREASED, URINE OUTPUT LESS THAN
400 ML PER DAY, URINE SEDIMENT BROAD CAST (S), URINE
SEDIMENT COARSE GRANULAR CAST (S), URINE SEDIMENT RBC,
```

```
URINE SEDIMENT RENAL TUBULAR CELL CAST (S), URINE
SEDIMENT WBC, WBC 4,000 TO 13,900 PERCENT NEUTRO-
PHIL (S) INCREASED, ELECTROPHORESIS SERUM ALBUMIN
DECREASED

DISCRIMINATE:  PROGRESSIVE SYSTEMIC SCLEROSIS
INVOLVING KIDNEYS, GLOMERULONEPHRITIS ADVANCED CHRONIC
```

(No positive information and no telling negative information has been received. The problem remains the same. The computer is arbitrarily programmed to a brief series of questions of a given class and then recalculates.)

```
URINE SEDIMENT FATTY CAST (S)?
NO

URINE SEDIMENT FAT BODIES?
NO
```

(The presence of fatty casts or fat bodies would favor chronic glomerulonephritis.)

```
PLEASE ENTER FINDINGS OF URINALYSIS OSMOLALITY AND
ELECTROLYTE (S)
*OMIT
```

("OMIT" means that no information is available about this group of items.)

```
URINE SEDIMENT WBS CAST (S)?
NO
```

(This is a weakly discriminating question. Its asking indicates that the system has exhausted *simple* discriminating questions.)

```
DISREGARDING:  WEIGHT INCREASE RECENT HX, BACK PAIN
SEVERE, DYSPNEA EXERTIONAL, ORTHOPNEA, ABDOMEN TENDER-
NESS RIGHT LOWER QUADRANT, CHEST PERCUSSION DULL
LOCALIZED, HAND (S) XRAY CONGENITAL SKELETAL
DEFECT (S), HEART MURMUR SYSTOLIC SECOND LEFT INTER-
SPACE, HEART SOUND (S) S2 SPLITTING WIDE AND FIXED,
HEART SOUND (S) S3 LEFT VENTRICULAR GALLOP, PULSE (S)
RADIAL DECREASED, RALES LOCALIZED, BICARBONATE BLOOD
LESS THAN 20, CHEST XRAY PLEURAL EFFUSION (S), CHEST
XRAY VASCULAR MARKING (S) INCREASED DIFFUSE, EKG
HEART BLOCK FIRST DEGREE, HEART XRAY LEFT ATRIUM
ENLARGED MODERATE, HEART XRAY MAIN PULMONARY ARTERY
ENLARGED, PHOSPHATE BLOOD INCREASED, RBC SCHIZOCYTE
```

```
(S) NUMEROUS, UREA NITROGEN BLOOD GTR THAN 100, FACTOR
VIII ANTIHEMOPHILIC INCREASED, FIBRINOGEN DEGRADATION
PRODUCT (S) BLOOD GTR THAN 25 MCG PER ML, HAPTOGLOBIN
PLASMA DECREASED, HEART ECHOCARDIOGRAPHY LEFT VENTRI-
CLE END-DIASTOLIC INTERNAL DIAMETER GTR THAN 5.6 CM,
HEART ECHOCARDIOGRAPHY RIGHT VENTRICLE END-DIASTOLIC
INTERNAL DIAMETER GTR THAN 2.3 CM, HEART ECHOCARDIOG-
RAPHY VENTRICULAR SEPTUM PARADOXIC SYSTOLIC MOTION,
LUNG (S) FEV1 DECREASED, LUNG (S) FORCED VITAL CAPAC-
ITY DECREASED, RBC RETICULOCYTE (S) GTR THAN 5 PER-
CENT, LUNG (S) RESIDUAL VOLUME INCREASED

CONSIDERING:  AGE 26 TO 55, CONTRACEPTIVE ORAL ADMIN-
ISTRATIVE RECENT HX, HYPERTENSION ABRUPT ONSET, SEX
FEMALE, BACK TENDERNESS COSTOVERTEBRAL ANGLE (S),
LEG (S) EDEMA BILATERAL SLIGHT OR MODERATE, PRESSURE
ARTERIAL DIASTOLIC GTR THAN 125, CREATININE BLOOD
INCREASED, HEART XRAY LEFT VENTRICLE ENLARGED,
HEMATOCRIT BLOOD LESS THAN 35, PROTEINURIA, UREA
NITROGEN BLOOD 30 TO 59, UREA NITROGEN BLOOD 60 TO
100, URIC ACID BLOOD INCREASED, URINE OUTPUT LESS THAN
400 ML PER DAY, URINE SEDIMENT BROAD CAST (S), URINE
SEDIMENT COARSE GRANULAR CAST (S), URINE SEDIMENT RBC,
URINE SEDIMENT RENAL TUBULAR CELL CAST (S), URINE
SEDIMENT WBC, WBC 4,000 TO 13,900 PERCENT NEUTRO-
PHIL (S) INCREASED, ELECTROPHORESIS SERUM ALBUMIN
DECREASED

DISCRIMINATE:  PROGRESSIVE SYSTEMIC SCLEROSIS INVOLV-
ING KIDNEYS, GLOMERULONEPHRITIS ADVANCED CHRONIC
```

(Having no further simple discriminating questions, the computer now turns to the LAB 2 category, inquiring about kidney biopsy, which is an invasive procedure. Interestingly, it has come to the same end point as did the patient's physicians. A renal biopsy was done to elucidate the nature of the kidney disease. The positive findings are entered as well as one negative observation.)

```
PLEASE ENTER FINDINGS OF KIDNEY BIOPSY

*KIDNEY BIOPSY ONION SKIN LESION (S) INTERLOBULAR
   ARTERY (IES)

*KIDNEY BIOPSY ARTERIOLAR ENDOTHELIAL PROLIFERATION

*KIDNEY BIOPSY GLOMERULI BASEMENT MEMBRANE THICKENING

*KIDNEY BIOPSY GLOMERULI PROLIFERATION CELL (S)

*KIDNEY BIOPSY INTERSTITIAL INFLAMMATION
```

*DENY

-KIDNEY BIOPSY GLOMERULI ANTIGEN ANTIBODY COMPLEX (ES)

-AFFIRM

*GO

DISREGARDING: WEIGHT INCREASE RECENT HX, BACK PAIN
SEVERE, DYSPNEA EXERTIONAL, ORTHOPNEA, ABDOMEN TENDER-
NESS RIGHT LOWER QUADRANT, CHEST PERCUSSION DULL
LOCALIZED, HAND (S) XRAY CONGENITAL SKELETAL DE-
FECT (S), HEART MURMUR SYSTOLIC SECOND LEFT INTER-
SPACE, HEART SOUND (S) S2 SPLITTING WIDE AND FIXED,
HEART SOUND (S) S3 LEFT VENTRICULAR GALLOP, PULSE (S)
RADIAL DECREASED, RALES LOCALIZED, BICARBONATE BLOOD
LESS THAN 20, CHEST XRAY PLEURAL EFFUSION (S), CHEST
XRAY VASCULAR MARKING (S) INCREASED DIFFUSE, EKG HEART
BLOCK FIRST DEGREE, HEART XRAY LEFT ATRIUM ENLARGED
MODERATE, HEART XRAY MAIN PULMONARY ARTERY ENLARGED,
PHOSPHATE BLOOD INCREASED, RBC SCHIZOCYTE (S) NUMER-
OUS, UREA NITROGEN BLOOD GTR THAN 100, FACTOR VIII
ANTIHEMOPHILIC INCREASED, FIBRINOGEN DEGRADATION
PRODUCT (S) BLOOD GTR THAN 25 MCG PER ML, HAPTOGLOBIN
PLASMA DECREASED, HEART ECHOCARDIOGRAPHY LEFT ATRIUM
INTERNAL DIAMETER 4 TO 6 CM, HEART ECHOCARDIOGRAPHY
LEFT VENTRICLE END-DIASTOLIC INTERNAL DIAMETER GTR
THAN 5.6 CM, HEART ECHOCARDIOGRAPHY RIGHT VENTRICLE
END-DIASTOLIC INTERNAL DIAMETER GTR THAN 2.3 CM, HEART
ECHOCARDIOGRAPHY VENTRICULAR SEPTUM PARADOXIC SYSTOLIC
MOTION, LUNG (S) FEV1 DECREASED, LUNG (S) FORCED VITAL
CAPACITY DECREASED, RBC RETICULOCYTE (S) GTR THAN
5 PERCENT, LUNG (S) RESIDUAL VOLUME INCREASED

CONSIDERING: AGE 26 TO 55, CONTRACEPTIVE ORAL ADMIN-
ISTRATION RECENT HX, HYPERTENSION ABRUPT ONSET, SEX
FEMALE, BACK TENDERNESS COSTOVERTEBRAL ANGLE (S),
LEG (S) EDEMA BILATERAL SLIGHT OR MODERATE, PRESSURE
ARTERIAL DIASTOLIC GTR THAN 125, CREATININE BLOOD
INCREASED, HEART XRAY LEFT VENTRICLE ENLARGED,
HEMATOCRIT BLOOD LESS THAN 35, PROTEINURIA, UREA
NITROGEN BLOOD 30 TO 59, UREA NITROGEN BLOOD 60 TO
100, URIC ACID BLOOD INCREASED, URINE OUTPUT LESS THAN
400 ML PER DAY, URINE SEDIMENT BROAD CAST (S), URINE
SEDIMENT COARSE GRANULAR CAST (S), URINE SEDIMENT RBC,
URINE SEDIMENT RENAL TUBULAR CELL CAST (S), URINE
SEDIMENT WBC, WBC 4,000 TO 13,900 PERCENT NEUTRO-
PHIL (S) INCREASED, ELECTROPHORESIS SERUM ALBUMIN
DECREASED, KIDNEY BIOPSY ARTERIOLAR ENDOTHELIAL PRO-
LIFERATION, KIDNEY BIOPSY GLOMERULI BASEMENT MEMBRANE
THICKENING, KIDNEY BIOPSY GLOMERULI PROLIFERATION
CELL (S), KIDNEY BIOPSY INTERSTITIAL INFLAMMATION,

```
KIDNEY BIOPSY ONION SKIN LESION (S) INTERLOBULAR
ARTERY (IES)

PURSUING:   PROGRESSIVE SYSTEMIC SCLEROSIS INVOLVING
    KIDNEYS
```

(The biopsy findings, particularly the onionskin lesions, support PSS involving the kidneys, and thus the system moves into the *Pursue* mode, indicating that it now has strong evidence for one diagnosis and will try to clinch it. A question is asked about an even more exclusive and almost pathognomonic biopsy finding in renal PSS. Renal arteriography was not performed, although there are some quite distinctive findings in renal PSS.)

```
KIDNEY BIOPSY INTERLOBULAR ARTERY (IES) ADVENTITIAL
FIBROSIS?
NO

PLEASE ENTER FINDINGS OF ARTERIOGRAPHY KIDNEY (S)
*OMIT

DISREGARDING: WEIGHT INCREASE RECENT HX, BACK PAIN
SEVERE, DYSPNEA EXERTIONAL, ORTHOPNEA, ABDOMEN TENDER-
NESS RIGHT LOWER QUADRANT, CHEST PERCUSSION DULL
LOCALIZED, HAND (S) XRAY CONGENITAL SKELETAL
DEFECT (S), HEART MURMUR SYSTOLIC SECOND LEFT INTER-
SPACE, HEART SOUND (S) S2 SPLITTING WIDE AND FIXED,
HEART SOUND (S) S3 LEFT VENTRICULAR GALLOP, PULSE (S)
RADIAL DECREASED, RALES LOCALIZED, BICARBONATE BLOOD
LESS THAN 20, CHEST XRAY PLEURAL EFFUSION (S), CHEST
XRAY VASCULAR MARKING (S) INCREASED DIFFUSE, EKG HEART
BLOCK FIRST DEGREE, HEART XRAY LEFT ATRIUM ENLARGED
MODERATE, HEART XRAY MAIN PULMONARY ARTERY ENLARGED,
PHOSPHATE BLOOD INCREASED, RBC SCHIZOCYTE (S) NUMER-
OUS, UREA NITROGEN BLOOD GTR THAN 100, FACTOR VIII
ANTIHEMOPHILIC INCREASED, FIBRINOGEN DEGRADATION
PRODUCT (S) BLOOD GTR THAN 25 MCG PER ML, HAPTOGLOBIN
PLASMA DECREASED, HEART ECHOCARDIOGRAPHY LEFT ATRIUM
INTERNAL DIAMETER 4 TO 6 CM, HEART ECHOCARDIOGRAPHY
LEFT VENTRICLE END-DIASTOLIC INTERNAL DIAMETER GTR
THAN 5.6 CM, HEART ECHOCARDIOGRAPHY RIGHT VENTRICLE
END-DIASTOLIC INTERNAL DIAMETER GTR THAN 2.3 CM, HEART
ECHOCARDIOGRAPHY VENTRICULAR SEPTUM PARADOXIC SYSTOLIC
MOTION, LUNG (S) FEV1 DECREASED, LUNG (S) FORCED VITAL
CAPACITY DECREASED, RBC RETICULOCYTE (S) GTR THAN
5 PERCENT, LUNG (S) RESIDUAL VOLUME INCREASED

CONSIDERING:   AGE 26 TO 55, CONTRACEPTIVE ORAL ADMIN-
ISTRATION RECENT HX, HYPERTENSION ABRUPT ONSET, SEX
FEMALE, BACK TENDERNESS COSTOVERTEBRAL ANGLE (S),
```

```
LEG (S) EDEMA BILATERAL SLIGHT OR MODERATE, PRESSURE
ARTERIAL DIASTOLIC GTR THAN 125, CREATININE BLOOD
INCREASED, HEART XRAY LEFT VENTRICLE ENLARGED,
HEMATOCRIT BLOOD LESS THAN 35, PROTEINURIA, UREA
NITROGEN BLOOD 30 TO 59, UREA NITROGEN BLOOD 60 TO
100, URIC ACID BLOOD INCREASED, URINE OUTPUT LESS THAN
400 ML PER DAY, URINE SEDIMENT BROAD CAST (S), URINE
SEDIMENT COARSE GRANULAR CAST (S), URINE SEDIMENT RBC,
URINE SEDIMENT RENAL TUBULAR CELL CAST (S), URINE
SEDIMENT WBC, WBC 4,000 TO 13,900 PERCENT NEUTRO-
PHIL (S) INCREASED, ELECTROPHORESIS SERUM ALBUMIN
DECREASED, KIDNEY BIOPSY ARTERIOLAR ENDOTHELIAL PRO-
LIFERATION, KIDNEY BIOPSY GLOMERULI BASEMENT MEMBRANE
THICKENING, KIDNEY BIOPSY GLOMERULI PROLIFERATION
CELL (S), KIDNEY BIOPSY INTERSTITIAL INFLAMMATION,
KIDNEY BIOPSY ONION SKIN LESION (S) INTERLOBULAR
ARTERY (IES)

PURSUING:   PROGRESSIVE SYSTEMIC SCLEROSIS INVOLVING
      KIDNEYS
CONCLUDE:   PROGRESSIVE SYSTEMIC SCLEROSIS INVOLVING
      KIDNEYS
```

(In spite of no further positive information, the system concludes PSS involving the kidneys; it had no reasonable competitor, given the data presented. The attempt to obtain further strengthening information indicates the conservative fashion in which the program is built.)

```
DISREGARDING:   BACK PAIN SEVERE, ABDOMEN TENDERNESS
RIGHT LOWER QUADRANT, HAND (S) XRAY CONGENITAL
SKELETAL DEFECT (S), HEART MURMUR SYSTOLIC SECOND LEFT
INTERSPACE, HEART SOUND (S) S2 SPLITTING WIDE AND
FIXED PULSE (S) RADIAL DECREASED, BICARBONATE BLOOD
LESS THAN 20, EKG HEART BLOCK FIRST DEGREE, HEART XRAY
LEFT ATRIUM ENLARGED MODERATE, HEART XRAY MAIN PULMO-
NARY ARTERY ENLARGED, PHOSPHATE BLOOD INCREASED, RBC
SCHIZOCYTE (S) NUMEROUS, UREA NITROGEN BLOOD GTR THAN
100, FACTOR VIII ANTIHEMOPHILIC INCREASED, FIBRINOGEN
DEGRADATION PRODUCT (S) BLOOD GTR THAN 25 MCG PER ML,
HAPTOGLOBIN PLASMA DECREASED, HEART ECHOCARDIOGRAPHY
RIGHT VENTRICLE END-DIASTOLIC INTERNAL DIAMETER GTR
THAN 2.3 GM, HEART ECHOCARDIOGRAPHY VENTRICULAR SEPTUM
PARADOXIC SYSTOLIC MOTION, LUNG (S) FEV1 DECREASED,
RBC RETICULOCYTE (S) GTR THAN 5 PERCENT, LUNG (S)
RESIDUAL VOLUME INCREASED

CONSIDERING:   WEIGHT INCREASE RECENT HX, DYSPNEA
EXERTIONAL, ORTHOPNEA, CHEST PERCUSSION DULL LOCAL-
IZED, HEART SOUND (S) S3 LEFT VENTRICULAR GALLOP,
RALES LOCALIZED, CHEST XRAY PLEURAL EFFUSION (S),
CHEST XRAY VASCULAR MARKING (S) INCREASED DIFFUSE,
```

```
HEART ECHOCARDIOGRAPHY LEFT ATRIUM INTERNAL DIAMETER
4 TO 6 CM, HEART ECHOCARDIOGRAPHY LEFT VENTRICLE END-
DIASTOLIC INTERNAL DIAMETER GTR THAN 5.6 CM, LUNG (S)
FORCED VITAL CAPACITY DECREASED

CONCLUDE:   CARDIAC FAILURE LEFT CHRONIC CONGESTIVE
```

(The system now reexamines the "disregarding" list, those manifestations not explained by renal PSS. It finds adequate evidence for congestive left heart failure and concludes that diagnosis. PSS involving the kidneys is "linked" to both acute and chronic left heart failure. Some clinicians might argue that the heart failure is subacute rather than chronic; in any case it is not truly acute.)

```
DISREGARDING:   BACK PAIN SEVERE, ABDOMEN TENDERNESS
RIGHT LOWER QUADRANT, PULSE (S) RADIAL DECREASED,
BICARBONATE BLOOD LESS THAN 20, HEART XRAY LEFT ATRIUM
ENLARGED MODERATE, PHOSPHATE BLOOD INCREASED, RBC
SCHIZOCYTE (S) NUMEROUS, UREA NITROGEN BLOOD GTR THAN
100, FACTOR VIII ANTIHEMOPHILIC INCREASED, FIBRINOGEN
DEGRADATION PRODUCT (S) BLOOD GTR THAN 25 MCG PER ML,
HAPTOGLOBIN PLASMA DECREASED, LUNG (S) FEV1 DECREASED,
RBC RETICULOCYTE (S) GTR THAN 5 PERCENT, LUNG (S)
RESIDUAL VOLUME INCREASED

CONSIDERING:   HEART MURMUR HX, HAND (S) XRAY CON-
GENITAL SKELETAL DEFECT (S), HEART MURMUR SYSTOLIC
SECOND LEFT INTERSPACE, HEART SOUND (S) S2 SPLITTING
WIDE AND FIXED, EKG HEART BLOCK FIRST DEGREE, HEART
XRAY MAIN PULMONARY ARTERY ENLARGED, HEART ECHO-
CARDIOGRAPHY RIGHT VENTRICLE END-DIASTOLIC INTERNAL
DIAMETER GTR THAN 2.3 CM, HEART ECHOCARDIOGRAPHY
VENTRICULAR SEPTUM PARADOXIC SYSTOLIC MOTION

PURSUING:   ATRIAL SEPTAL DEFECT

PLEASE ENTER FINDINGS OF ECHOGRAM HEART AND GREAT
     VESSEL (S)
*GO

HEART ECHOCARDIOGRAPHY TRICUSPID VALVE LEAFLET (S)
     DIASTOLIC FLUTTER?
N/A

PLEASE ENTER FINDINGS OF ANGIOCARDIOGRAPHY
*OMIT

PLEASE ENTER FINDINGS OF CARDIAC CATHETERIZATION
*OMIT

CONCLUDE:   ATRIAL SEPTAL DEFECT
```

(The system has now focused attention on a disorder totally unrelated to the diagnoses already made. The patient did have this form of congenital heart disease. Once again in a conservative way, the system tries to obtain additional suportive data, but, getting none, it considers the information already available to be conclusive.)

```
DISREGARDING:  BACK PAIN SEVERE, ABDOMEN TENDERNESS
RIGHT LOWER QUADRANT, PULSE (S) RADIAL DECREASED,
HEART XRAY LEFT ATRIUM ENLARGED MODERATE, RBC
SCHIZOCYTE (S) NUMEROUS, FACTOR VIII ANTIHEMOPHILIC
INCREASED, FIBRINOGEN DEGRADATION PRODUCT (S) BLOOD
GTR THAN 25 MCG PER ML, HAPTOGLOBIN PLASMA DECREASED,
LUNG (S) FEV1 DECREASED, RBC RETICULOCYTE (S) GTR THAN
5 PERCENT, LUNG (S) RESIDUAL VOLUME INCREASED

CONSIDERING:  BICARBONATE BLOOD LESS THAN 20,
PHOSPHATE BLOOD INCREASED, UREA NITROGEN BLOOD GTR
THAN 100, BLEEDING TIME INCREASED

DISCRIMINATE:  RENAL FAILURE ACUTE, RENAL FAILURE
CHRONIC (UREMIA)

AZOTEMIA TWO WEEK (S) DURATION OR LESS?
YES

PLEASE ENTER FINDINGS FOR FECES EXAM ROUTINE
*GO

FECES GROSS BLOOD?
NO

BREATH URINIFEROUS?
N/A

DISREGARDING:  BACK PAIN SEVERE, ABDOMEN TENDERNESS
RIGHT LOWER QUADRANT, PULSE (S) RADIAL DECREASED,
HEART XRAY LEFT ATRIUM ENLARGED MODERATE, RBC
SCHIZOCYTE (S) NUMEROUS, FACTOR VIII ANTIHEMOPHILIC
INCREASED, FIBRINOGEN DEGRADATION PRODUCT (S) BLOOD
GTR THAN 25 MCG PER ML, HAPTOGLOBIN PLASMA DECREASED,
LUNG (S) FEV1 DECREASED, RBC RETICULOCYTE (S) GTR THAN
5 PERCENT, LUNG (S) RESIDUAL VOLUME INCREASED

CONSIDERING:  AZOTEMIA TWO WEEK (S) DURATION OR LESS,
BICARBONATE BLOOD LESS THAN 20, PHOSPHATE BLOOD
INCREASED, UREA NITROGEN BLOOD GTR THAN 100, BLEEDING
TIME INCREASED

PURSUING:  RENAL FAILURE ACUTE
CONCLUDE:  RENAL FAILURE ACUTE
```

(The diagnosis of acute renal failure presents no problem once the duration of azotemia is known.)

```
DISREGARDING:  ABDOMEN TENDERNESS RIGHT LOWER QUAD-
RANT, PULSE (S) RADIAL DECREASED, HEART XRAY LEFT
ATRIUM ENLARGED MODERATE, LUNG (S) FEV1 DECREASED,
LUNG (S) RESIDUAL VOLUME INCREASED

CONSIDERING:  BACK PAIN SEVERE, RBC SCHIZOCYTE (S)
NUMEROUS, FACTOR VIII ANTIHEMOPHILIC INCREASED,
FIBRINOGEN DEGRADATION PRODUCT (S) BLOOD GTR THAN
25 MCG PER ML, HAPTOGLOBIN PLASMA DECREASED, LDH BLOOD
INCREASED, RBC RETICULOCYTE (S) GTR THAN 5 PERCENT

PURSUING:  DISSEMINATED INTRAVASCULAR COAGULATION
ACUTE

PLEASE ENTER FINDINGS OF OBSTETRICAL STATUS/HX
*GO

PREGNANCY CURRENT BY HX OR PELVIC EXAM?
NO


DISREGARDING:  ABDOMEN TENDERNESS RIGHT LOWER QUAD-
RANT PULSE (S) RADIAL DECREASED, HEART XRAY LEFT
ATRIUM ENLARGED MODERATE, LUNG (S) FEV1 DECREASED,
LUNG (S) RESIDUAL VOLUME INCREASED

CONSIDERING:  BACK PAIN SEVERE, RBC SCHIZOCYTE (S)
NUMEROUS, FACTOR VIII ANTIHEMOPHILIC INCREASED,
FIBRINOGEN DEGRADATION PRODUCT (S) BLOOD GTR THAN
25 MCG PER ML, HAPTOGLOBIN PLASMA DECREASED, LDH BLOOD
INCREASED, RBC RETICULOCYTE (S) GTR THAN 5 PERCENT

PURSUING:  DISSEMINATED INTRAVASCULAR COAGULATION
ACUTE

PLEASE ENTER FINDINGS OF COAGULATION TEST (S)
*GO

ANTITHROMBIN III LESS THAN 50 PERCENT OF NORMAL?
N/A

ETHANOL GEL TEST POSITIVE?
N/A

PROTAMINE PARACOAGULATION TEST POSITIVE?
N/A

BLOOD INCOAGULABLE?
NO
```

```
FACTOR V PROACCELERIN DECREASED?
N/A

FIBRINOGEN BLOOD DECREASED?
N/A

DISREGARDING: ABDOMEN TENDERNESS RIGHT LOWER QUAD-
RANT, PULSE (S) RADIAL DECREASED, HEART XRAY LEFT
ATRIUM ENLARGED MODERATE, LUNG (S) FEV1 DECREASED,
LUNG (S) RESIDUAL VOLUME INCREASED

CONSIDERING: BACK PAIN SEVERE, RBC SCHIZOCYTE (S)
NUMEROUS, FACTOR VIII ANTIHEMOPHILIC INCREASED,
FIBRINOGEN DEGRADATION PRODUCT (S) BLOOD GTR THAN
25 MCG PER ML, HAPTOGLOBIN PLASMA DECREASED, LDH BLOOD
INCREASED, RBC RETICULOCYTE (S) GTR THAN 5 PERCENT

PURSUING: DISSEMINATED INTRAVASCULAR COAGULATION
ACUTE
CONCLUDE: DISSEMINATED INTRAVASCULAR COAGULATION
ACUTE
```

(This complication of the patient's severe illness is correctly diagnosed. Again, some of the expected blood coagulation abnormalities
are sought after, but not being known about (N/A), the evidence is
considered conclusive.

The reader should note the items remaining on the "disregarding"
list. The decreased radial pulse is the only immediate evidence for
systemic sclerosis or scleroderma. The alterations in pulmonary function suggest pulmonary fibrosis secondary to PSS. The program will
deal with these considerations but in the absence of additional information cannot be conclusive.)

It must be emphasized that this program in computer-assisted diagnosis is still at the stage of research and development. It is evident
there are a number of problems with the program. The diagnostic
process is a sequential one. It must be concluded that the patient has
disease A before the strengths between A and B are brought into force.
The clinician often does not use a sequential format. Instead it is
postulated that the patient has disease A plus B from the beginning.
The program has a weak time axis. Time can be dealt with partly
through the mode of questioning, but the system does not adequately
deal with the time factor in the evolution of disease. The program
favors common disease, a fact which has advantages and disadvantages. As pointed out, the physician does that too; but when the
differential diagnosis involves the individual patient who has a rare

disorder, the system may favor a common disease over it. And the program also favors systemic diseases, multisystem diseases that explain many, many things. Sometimes such a conclusion is correct, but at other times the patient has a combination of illnesses instead of one complex disease, and the program tends to favor the complex one. Certain practical considerations, mentioned earlier, such as the emergency nature of an illness, are not dealt with. So there are plenty of problems remaining in this process, but in further devising it is our intention to try to follow the principles and the process of human diagnosis. In that sense the computer program is an empirical system. In fact, Dr. Pople first built it by putting me through what I have always called a diagnostic psychoanalysis. I analyzed many cases for him, he saw the principles involved, and that was the basis for INTERNIST-I.

REFERENCES

Miller, R., H. Pople and J. Myers. 1982. INTERNIST-I, an experimental computer-based diagnostic consultant for general internal medicine. *New England Journal of Medicine* 307:468–476.

Scully, R., ed. 1978. Case records of the Massachusetts General Hospital. *New England Journal of Medicine* 299:466–474.

9

Coming to Grips with the Multiple-Diagnosis Problem

Harry E. Pople, Jr.

Diagnosis in internal medicine is frequently complicated by the need to discern multiple diseases in a single patient. In order to enable computer-based diagnostic systems to deal with such complex clinical problems, it is necessary to devise problem-formation heuristics that can effectively partition the set of disease hypotheses evoked by a given set of clinical manifestations into coherent subsets, within which diagnostic problem-solving methods may be applied. One such system, referred to as INTERNIST, is being developed in our laboratory at the University of Pittsburgh. My principal medical collaborator in this work has been Jack D. Myers, M.D., University Professor of Medicine at Pittsburgh.

Because INTERNIST is intended to serve a consulting role in medical diagnosis, it has been challenged with a wide variety of difficult clinical problems: cases published in the medical journals, clinical pathological conferences, other interesting and unusual problems arising in the local teaching hospitals. In the great majority of these test cases, the problem-formation strategy of INTERNIST has proved to be effective in sorting out the pieces of the puzzle and coming to a correct diagnosis, involving in some cases as many as a dozen disease entities.

My purpose today will be to discuss the problem-formation heuristic underpinning this performance of INTERNIST and to share with you our current thinking with regard to this important aspect of clinical decision making.

BACKGROUND

First, let me clarify what I mean by the term *problem*. For present purposes this term is taken to mean a collection of disease entities, one and only one of which is considered possible in the case being studied. In many computer-based diagnostic systems, the "problem" (so defined) is predetermined, and the program's job is simply to select from a fixed list of disease entities one that best fits the facts of a case.

A diagnostic program based on Bayes' rule, for example, requires that the problems of differential diagnosis be defined as sets of disease entities which (sets) are exhaustive (i.e., all possibilities are included) and consist of mutually exclusive disease entities (i.e., one and only one may occur) [1–3].

There are both philosophical and methodological problems associated with the use of Bayes' rule in medical diagnosis; these have been well documented in the literature [4–6]. A major problem is the need to assume that the manifestations of disease are statistically independent so as to reduce the data-structuring problem to manageable proportions. A second problem, which bears on the multiple-disease issue, is the requirement that for purposes of Bayesian analysis, the set of possible diagnoses must be exhaustive and mutually exclusive.

In order to deal with complex clinical problems having the potential of multiple diagnoses, some authors have proposed the development of diagnostic programs comprising sets of integrated Bayesian procedures, each dealing with some well-defined subproblem in clinical medicine. Thus the set of all disease entities would be divided into M subsets, not necessarily disjoint, each of which constitutes a mutually exclusive and exhaustive "differential diagnosis" list. If M is a relatively small number, it may be feasible to employ a Bayesian decision procedure that attempts to solve all M decision problems simultaneously [7, 8]. Alternatively, one may invoke heuristic "activation rules" or rely upon the guidance of persons using the system to select appropriate subproblems for further analysis [9, 10]. As this latter approach requires that an initial decision be made concerning the subproblems to be explored, great care must be taken to ensure that the analytical process has the capacity to recover from "false starts."

Otherwise, the types of difficulties often encountered in branching-logic diagnostic systems, discussed in the following paragraph, may limit the usefulness of this approach. We shall return to consideration of this important issue again during the discussion of INTERNIST-II (see below, "Concurrent Problem-Formation in INTERNIST-II").

Aside from Bayesian methods, the other approach to computer-based diagnosis that has been most extensively studied is the "branching-logic" or "flowchart" method. The essence of this approach is the use of a sequence of discriminating questions that successively narrow the diagnostic possibilities that may be considered for a case under analysis, until ultimately in the limiting case some single diagnosis remains.

Behaviorally, a diagnostic procedure using branching logic would appear to perform in much the same manner as a sequential Bayesian procedure [11, 12]. There are, however, major differences in the forms of the data base and in the inference procedures that are employed.

The data base for a branching-logic procedure is a network, each node of which represents a decision (interrogation) point. Depending on the given initial conditions of a case, the inferential procedure begins at some starting point of the network and then proceeds from node to node, eliciting at each point the discriminating information required by the decision process associated with the node. A decision is then made, on the basis of this result, as to which node is to be considered next. (See figure 1.)

The major drawback of this method has been its inability to handle new and conflicting information after several previous decisions have been made. As the focus of attention moves through the net, previous nodes or decisions become inaccessible, rendering it impossible to retreat from a given pathway under the influence of new information. In essence the model under certain circumstances may find itself "out on a limb" from which it cannot extricate itself.

Another deficiency of this method is that, unlike the Bayesian procedure described earlier and the INTERNIST approach to be discussed later, a diagnostic program based on branching logic is not capable of processing input data presented in random order. The sequence of information inputs required in the course of a diagnostic study is completely determined by the structure of the decision network and by the sequence of prior decisions made along the way.

These characteristics of the branching-logic method preclude its use as a general clinical diagnostic tool. The method has, however, proved

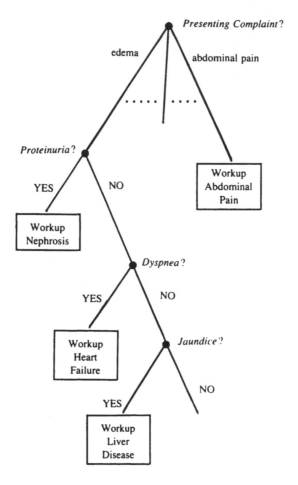

Figure 1. Branching Logic Approach to Diagnosis

to be extremely useful in certain phases of the diagnostic process—for example, the staging and analysis of laboratory test data [13].

AN ARTIFICIAL-INTELLIGENCE APPROACH
TO MEDICAL DIAGNOSIS

Several major investigations have been undertaken during the past few years, seeking to apply the methods of artificial intelligence to problems of medical diagnosis and management. In our own work the emphasis has been on development of a computer-based diagnostic system for internal medicine. Other studies have focused on the diagnosis and therapeutic management of bacteremia [14], the differential diagnosis of glaucoma [15], the management of digitalis therapy [16], and the taking of the present illness [17].

Development of the system which we now call INTERNIST-I was begun about seven years ago. The system was successfully demonstrated for the first time in 1974 and has been used since that time in the analysis of hundreds of clinical problems.

This system employs a novel attention-focusing heuristic in order to deal sequentially with the component parts of a complex clinical problem. In effect, the program composes dynamically—on the basis of evidence provided—what in context constitutes a subset of exhaustive and mutually exclusive disease entities that can explain some significant subset of the observed manifestations of disease. This heuristic process, which we refer to as "problem formation," is described more fully in the following section.

On the basis of extensive testing of this initial INTERNIST system, it has become clear that many aspects of the system's performance could be significantly improved if it were possible to deal with the various component problems and their interrelationships simultaneously. This has led to the development of INTERNIST-II, a system embodying strategies of concurrent problem-formation that we expect will yield more rapid convergence to the correct diagnosis in many cases, and in at least some cases provide more acceptable diagnostic behavior.

In the following section, the information structures and heuristic processes underlying performance of the INTERNIST-I system will be reviewed briefly (a more complete description can be found in Pople et al. [18]); this will be followed by a somewhat more detailed discussion of the methods employed in the formation and synthesis of composite hypotheses of INTERNIST-II.

THE INTERNIST KNOWLEDGE BASE

The knowledge base underlying both INTERNIST systems is composed of two basic types of elements: disease entities and manifestations (history items, symptoms, physical signs, laboratory data). In addition, there are a number of relations defined on these classes of elements. At present there are approximately five hundred disease entities encoded in the knowledge base and over three thousand manifestations.

Each disease entity had an associated list of manifestations known to occur in that disease, recorded along with an estimate on a scale of 1–5 of the frequency of occurrence. The inverse of this relation is also recorded explicitly in the knowledge base; thus, each manifestation is associated with the list of diseases in which the manifestation is known to occur, again with a weighting factor (in this case on a 0–5 scale) intended to reflect the strength of association. We refer to this weight as the "evoking strength" by which a manifestation is related to each disease on its "evokes-list."

There is also recorded a hierarchy of disease categories, organized primarily around the concept of organ systems, having at the top level such categories as "liver disease," "lung disease," "kidney disease," and so on. Each of these areas is divided into more specific categories, which may in turn be further subdivided any number of times until the terminal level representing individual disease entities is reached. The reason for including such a hierarchy of categories in the knowledge base is to make it possible to form hypotheses and conclusions concerning higher-level descriptions of disease process in cases where the data do not permit more precise judgments.

Other relations are defined on the set of disease entities to record the causal, temporal, and other patterns of association by which the various disease entities are interrelated. There are also several auxiliary relations defined on the class of manifestations to record properties of interest (such as the type and importance of a manifestation) and relations among manifestations (such as the derivability of one from another).

Problem-Formation Methods

As mentioned previously, for present purposes the term *problem* is taken to mean a collection of disease entities, one and only one of which is considered possible in the case being analyzed. Whereas, in many computer-based diagnostic systems the problem (so defined) is predetermined and the program's job is simply to select from a fixed list of disease entities the one that best fits the facts of the case, in cases where more than one disease may be present it is necessary to partition the set of disease entities evoked by a given set of observed manifestations into disjoint subsets. The approach taken in INTERNIST-I has been to focus on one problem at a time, with each successive problem dynamically determined by the facts of the case developed up to that point. The process is as follows:

First, disease entities that can explain any or all of the observed findings are weighed individually and assigned scores reflecting their goodness of fit with the data. In this scoring process, the "evoking strength" and "importance" of manifestations explained by a disease are counted in its favor; "frequency" weights count against those disease hypotheses in which the corresponding manifestations are expected but not found present in the case.

Given a ranked list of disease hypotheses, a problem is then formulated on the basis of the most highly rated of these items, using the following heuristic criterion: two disease entities are considered to be alternatives to one another (hence part of the same problem definition) if, taken together, they explain no more of the observed findings than are explained by one or the other separately.

The set of alternatives so determined, with scores within a fixed range of the top-ranked disease hypotheses on the list, are then composed into a problem that becomes the focus of problem-solving attention.

The program then selects questions that will help to discriminate among entities in the problem set, reevaluates all diseases evoked (whether in or out of the problem focus) on the basis of new information obtained, and then reformulates the problem focus. Depending on which disease entity emerges as most highly rated on successive iterations of the process, the focus of attention may shift from one problem to another—but at any one time there is a single problem under active consideration.

Whenever a problem becomes solved, it is entered into a list of concluded diagnoses; all manifestations explained by that disease are marked "accounted for"; and the process recycles until all problems present in the case have been uncovered.

As was pointed out earlier, because of causal, temporal, or other interrelationships certain combinations of disease entities are more likely to occur than others. This fact is recognized in INTERNIST-I by the scoring algorithm, which on each iteration of the process gives additional weight to any disease entity that is in any way linked to some already concluded disease.

Critique

Though exceedingly robust and proven effective in solving a wide range of difficult clinical problems, the sequential approach to problem formation and solution incorporated in INTERNIST-I is not without its shortcomings.

Monitoring the reactions of clinicians who have interacted with the system over the past three years has disclosed several major performance deficiencies. Of primary concern is the tendency of the program, in complex cases, to begin its analysis by considering wholly inappropriate problems, on which it may spend an inordinate amount of time. This rarely leads to a false conclusion but does prolong the sessions of terminal interaction unnecessarily. There are several reasons to account for this phenomenon, all of which are related to the system's inability to perceive the multiplicity of problems in a case all at once.

If, for example, it were possible to structure several problems at the same time, heuristics might be employed to focus problem-solving attention on the most "solvable" of these, rather than the one that happens to receive the highest goodness-of-fit rating as described above. Moreover, the scoring process itself could be made more effective if the findings of a case could be distributed among the several concurrent problem-areas in accordance with some notion of relevancy. At present, lacking the perspective of a multiple-problem focus, IN-TERNIST-I assigns credit in the scoring of a disease hypothesis to all manifestations explained by that disease, however rare that association. Hence in a case, say, involving obvious liver and gastrointestinal involvement, the singular focus of INTERNIST-I will invariably favor those liver problems that also generate gastrointestinal findings and those gastrointestinal disorders that give rise to what are predominantly liver manifestations. The clinician, able to recognize that both problem areas are involved, can attribute findings to the most relevant problem areas, thereby coming in many cases to a far better ranking of the alternatives in each subproblem. The clinician can also take prior cognizance of the interrelationships among disease entities in order to come more quickly to specific hypotheses than would otherwise be the case.

In summary, the design of INTERNIST-I was motivated by the need to formulate and focus attention on individual components of complex clinical problems. Experience with this system suggests, however, that a multiproblem focus and prior attention to the interrelationships among hypothesized disease entities might yield patterns of behavior that would appear more reasonable and hence more acceptable to the clinician users of the system. These observations set the stage for the design of the successor system described in the following section.

CONCURRENT PROBLEM-FORMATION IN INTERNIST-II

The "Constrictor" Concept

Clinicians have a term *pathognomonic* that refers to any manifestation distinctively characteristic of a particular disease; the occurrence of such a finding is sufficient to warrant the conclusion of the associated disease. Unfortunately, such pathognomonic associations between manifestations and disease entities are rare, and are by and large derived from special laboratory or invasive procedures that are expensive and/or dangerous for the patient. Hence, one cannot indiscriminately seek pathognomonic findings in order to enhance the problem-formation capability of a diagnostic problem.

We can, however, extend the concept of pathognomonic association to achieve a very useful tool for generation of multiple hypotheses. If the focus of attention is directed at higher levels of the disease hierarchy rather than at the terminal-level nodes, quite specific associations between very commonplace manifestations and these higher-level disease descriptors can often be established. For example, jaundice, which is a readily observed physical sign, is a reasonably strong cue that some problem within the general category of liver disease is present, although it provides virtually no help in further discrimination within this subarea. Similarly, bloody sputum, while not pathognomonic with respect to any particular lung problem, provides ample justification for serious consideration of the lung area as a problem focus.

The existence of these specific patterns of association between certain commonly observed manifestations and higher-level disease descriptors has led to the conjecture that the clinician's facility in delineating the multiproblem structure of a clinical case derives, at least in part, from his attention to what we have come to call the "constrictors" of a case—those individual findings or combinations of findings that strongly cue the hypothesizing of some unspecified problem within each of several categories of the disease hierarchy [19].

We have analyzed the pattern of constrictor relationships among manifestations and disease categories in the INTERNIST data base and have incorporated the resulting set of associations as an additional information structure accessible to the diagnostic programs. In reviewing the data, we found that while many manifestations are uniquely associated with particular high-level categories of the hierarchy, other associations are merely "predominant"; that is, though rare, the possibility exists of certain findings being explained in areas other than the one to which they have been assigned in the constrictor relation. As might be expected, the occurrence of strict constrictor associations becomes less frequent as one considers more specific disease categories, and by the time terminal nodes are reached, the constrictor relation is essentially limited to the pathognomonic manifestations.

Because constrictors come with varying degrees of certitude, it is important to recognize the heuristic nature of any multiproblem-formation strategy based on the concept. Hence, it is necessary to view the problem-formation process as conjectural, and to have provision for retreating from any multiple-problem hypothesis that might be adduced, in order to consider other alternatives.

The Multiproblem Generator

INTERNIST-II employs a hypothesis generator that uses the concept of constrictor to delineate the top-level structure of a complex problem, and a modified scoring algorithm that considers within each subproblem only those findings judged to be relevant in that context.

The process, briefly, is as follows: First, each evoked disease category is weighed on the basis of the importance of those observed manifestations explained by some disease in that category, with negative findings causing reductions in the score where appropriate. Then a multiple-problem generator is invoked to formulate what we refer to as the root structure of the overall problem. This generator constructs a conjunctive set of category hypotheses by selecting first on the basis of constrictor certitude, then on the basis of the score assigned to each area. A running record of unexplained findings is progressively reduced as successive hypotheses are entered into the root structure, and the generator eventually terminates when all findings have been covered by at least one hypothesis. Because this construction is a heuristic process, these generators are maintained in readiness, so that alternative root structures may be generated if called for at some later time.

The root-level hypotheses may or may not constitute "problems" in the technical sense that this term was used in the previous section. That is, there is no assurance that the conjecture of a problem within some high-level disease category makes reference to a single disease entity there. For example, cirrhosis of the liver and cirrhotic portal hypertension—both disease entities in the liver area—often co-occur in the same patient.

Thus the need exists for some method of refining the root-level hypothesis structures by the introduction of subproblem conjectures where appropriate. Provided that there are suitable constrictor cues in the data to justify such subdivision, the multiproblem generator just described can be employed in this hypothesis-reduction task.

There are obvious analogies that can be drawn between this hypothesis-formation-and-reduction procedure and the more familiar problem-solving methods employed in other "artificial-intelligence" applications [20]. What we have described is a search process (see figure 2), the goal of which is achievement of a state in which each subproblem is characterized by the presumption of a single disease occurrence (we refer to such a subproblem as a *simplex*). Note that in general a great many hypothesis states can be formulated so as to satisfy this "goal" criterion. Hence additional criteria and procedures must be devised to focus attention on the most useful formulation from among those satisfying the goal.

An important criterion that is often invoked in clinical decision making is that of Occam's razor. This is the maxim requiring that the simpler of competing hypotheses be preferred to the more complex. As interpreted in the practice of medical diagnosis, this rule adjures the clinician to seek, if possible, a unitary cause to account for all observed findings in a patient. This does not necessarily call for the identification of a single disease entity, as we have used this term previously. A unitary hypothesis can include a number of distinct entities interrelated via some pathophysiological (i.e., causal) mechanism.

In keeping with this principle of parsimony, we have developed a procedure by which separate simplex-problem specifications can be combined into a unitary *complex* hypothesis. This procedure, which we refer to as *synthesis,* can be thought of as a state-transformation

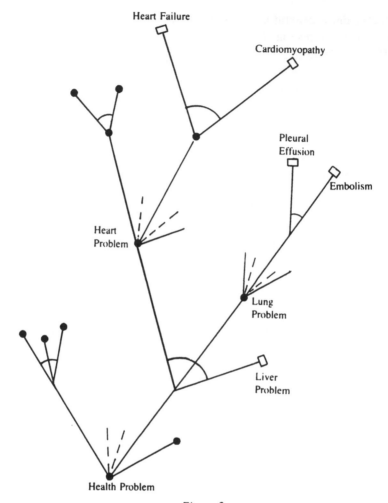

Figure 2.

operator that maps partially expanded hypothesis states into new states wherein two or more *simplex* nodes have been combined into a single *complex* node. The basis for such combinations is the existence of causal, temporal, or other known patterns of association among members of these simplex-problem sets.

By use of the synthesis procedure whenever a sufficiently strong simplex is adduced, the resolution of other related subproblems can be conjectured even in the absence of discriminating primary evidence. Thus, for example, if there is reasonably strong evidence that a patient has congestive heart failure and also some form of ascites, the strong link between heart failure and the transudative form of ascites can be invoked to resolve the ambiguity with respect to the latter problem.

The effect of the problem-formation and synthesis heuristics of INTERNIST-II is best illustrated by example. The case analysis presented below uses data from the clinical pathological conference published in the *New England Journal of Medicine* 290:1071. Several other published CPC's have also been tested with comparable results.

CASE ANALYSIS

The important diagnoses for this case included primary cardiomyopathy, congestive heart failure with plural effusion, transudative ascites, cardiac cirrhosis resulting from chronic hepatic congestion, and acute tubular necrosis of kidneys caused by caridogenic shock. There is also evidence of systemic embolism.

After initial findings are read in (see figure 3a), INTERNIST-II develops two multiproblem formulations, the first without use of the synthesis procedure (figure 3b) and the second using synthesis in the fashion described above (figure 3c). Both formulations are correct. It can readily be seen, however, that several of the simplex problems, viewed as independent entities, contain little in the way of discriminating data.

On the basis of perceived relationships between specific diseases of the several problem areas, the synthesis procedure of INTERNIST-II effectively narrows the problem focus. It should be emphasized, however, that this is a heuristic mechanism used solely to direct the future work-up of the case, not to render final decisions. It is important to bear in mind that particular clinical problems may involve two or more *independent* disease entities and that the imperative to develop unitary hypotheses is not always correct. Hence the hypothesis-formation-and-refinement process of INTERNIST-II is structured as a state-space search [21] within which it is possible to attend to the principle of parsimony, while reserving the option of retreating to alternative formulations when the evidence so requires.

OBSERVATIONS

The primary goal for INTERNIST-II has been to achieve a capability for concurrent problem-formation in order that improved scoring

```
AGE 26 TO 55
SEX MALE
DYSPNEA EXERTIONAL
HEART OUTPUT DECREASED
HEART CATHETERIZATION LEFT VENTRICLE END DIASTOLIC
    PRESSURE INCREASED
HEART FAILURE CONGESTIVE HX
PRESSURE ARTERIAL SYSTOLIC LESS THAN 90
THROMBOPHLEBITIS
LIVER ENLARGED MODERATE
EKG PREMATURE ATRIAL CONTRACTION (S)
EKG VENTRICULAR CONTRACTION (S)
EKG HEART BLOCK FIRST DEGREE
EKG LEFT BUNDLE BRANCH BLOCK
EKG LOW VOLTAGE
EKG ATRIAL FIBRILLATION
COUGH
TACHYCARDIA
PRESSURE VENOUS CENTRAL GTR THAN 10
PRESSURE VENOUS INCREASED INSPECTION
RHONCHI DIFFUSE
HEART SOUND (S) SUMMATION GALLOP LEFT VENTRICULAR
HEART PERCUSSION LEFT BORDER LATERAL DISPLACEMENT
HEART IMPULSE APICAL FORCEFUL
ABDOMEN TENDERNESS RIGHT UPPER QUADRANT
HEART XRAY LEFT VENTRICLE ENLARGEMENT
HEART XRAY RIGHT VENTRICLE ENLARGEMENT
WBC 14000 TO 30000
PLATELET (S) 50000 TO 200000
CHEST XRAY LUNG (S) CONGESTED
CHEST XRAY PLEURAL EFFUSION (S)
URINE OUTPUT LESS THAN 400 CC PER DAY
UREA NITROGEN BLOOD 30 TO 60
BILIRUBIN CONJUGATED BLOOD INCREASED
SGOT GTR THAN 400
LDH BLOOD INCREASED
CPK BLOOD INCREASED
ABDOMEN FLANK (S) BULGING BILATERAL
ABDOMEN FLANK (S) HEAVY BILATERAL
ABDOMEN DULLNESS SHIFTING
PROTHROMBIN TIME INCREASED
CALCIUM BLOOD DECREASED
PHOSPHATE BLOOD INCREASED
ELECTROPHORESIS SERUM ALBUMIN DECREASED
ALKALINE PHOSPHATASE INCREASED UP TO 2 TIMES NORMAL
URINE SEDIMENT RBC
```

Figure 3a. Manifestations Entered for Analysis

```
PROBLEM:
  CHYLOUS ASCITES 26
  EXUDATIVE ASCITES 16
  TRANSUDATIVE ASCITES 26
  ACUTE GENERALIZED PERITONITIS 12

PROBLEM:
  CHRONIC CONGESTIVE LEFT HEART FAILURE 185

PROBLEM:
  ALCOHOLIC HEPATITIS 116
  LEPTOSPIROSIS WITH HEPATIC INVOLVEMENT 112
  HEPATOCELLULAR CARCINOMA 111
  SECONDARY NEOPLASM OF THE LIVER 106
  ACUTE VIRAL HEPATITIS 106
  HEPATIC MILIARY TUBERCULOSIS 106
  CHRONIC ACTIVE HEPATITIS 106
  HODGKIN'S DISEASE OF THE LIVER 101
  DRUG HYPERSENSITIVITY HEPATOCELLULAR REACTION 100
  INFECTIOUS MONONUCLEOSIS 100
  HEPATIC CONGESTION 100
  HEPATIC POLYARTERITIS 100
  PRIMARY BILARY CIRRHOSIS 100
  ACUTE VIRAL HEPATITIS CHOLESTATIC TYPE 100

PROBLEM:
  EMPYEMA 56
  SECONDARY PULMONARY MALIGNANT NEOPLASM (LYMPHOGENOUS
    TYPE) 55
  HEMOTHORAX 50
  PLEURAL EFFUSION TRANSUDATE 46
  PLEURAL EFFUSION CHYLOUS 46
  PRIMARY BRONCHOGENIC CARCINOMA 42
  BRONCHIOLAR-ALVEOLAR CELL CARCINOMA 42
  PLEURAL EFFUSION EXUDATE 40

PROBLEM:
  ACUTE CARDIOGENIC SHOCK 158

PROBLEM:
  ACUTE MASSIVE PULMONARY EMBOLISM 92

PROBLEM:
  CARDIOMYOPATHY PRIMARY 144
  CARDIOMYOPATHY SECONDARY 130

PROBLEM;
  LEPTOSPIROSIS WITH RENAL INVOLVEMENT 82
  ACUTE TUBULAR NECROSIS 70

UNEXPLAINED:
  CALCIUM BLOOD DECREASED 3
```

Figure 3b. Problem Focus of INTERNIST-II Without Synthesis

```
SIMPLEX:
  ACUTE MASSIVE PULMONARY EMBOLISM
COMPLEX:
  ACUTE CARDIOGENIC SHOCK
  CAUSING
    ACUTE TUBULAR NECROSIS
COMPLEX:
  ONE OF THE FOLLOWING:
    CARDIOMYOPATHY PRIMARY
    CARDIOMYOPATHY SECONDARY
  CAUSING
    PLEURAL EFFUSION TRANSUDATE
  ALSO CAUSING
    TRANSUDATIVE ASCITES
  ALSO CAUSING
    HEPATIC CONGESTION
```

Figure 3c. Problem Focus of INTERNIST-II
Using Synthesis

methods and attention to the principle of parsimony may be exploited in the development of what will be perceived by clinicians to be reasonable problem conjectures.

At least in the development of initial problem formulations, early results suggest that we can expect performance surpassing that of predecessor systems. What remains to be seen is the adequacy of the state-space formalism as a framework within which appropriate reformulation of the problem set can be recognized and/or developed in those cases when the initial focus is, at least in part, incorrect.

SUMMARY

In this paper it has been argued that the more traditional approaches to computer-based medical diagnosis are inadequate to deal with the general problem of diagnosis in internal medicine. The reason for this is that in many cases, especially those requiring diagnostic consultation, patients can present with a number of concurrent clinical problems. In order to deal with such complex clinical problems we have found it necessary to devise problem-formation heuristics that can effectively partition the set of disease hypotheses evoked by a given set of clinical manifestations into coherent subsets, within which diagnostic problem-solving methods may be applied.

Two approaches to this problem have been described, one dealing with sequential problem formation and solution, the other emphasizing concurrent consideration of the component parts of complex clinical problems.

One of the great strengths of INTERNIST-I is its ability to shift the focus of attention from one problem to another on the basis of newly derived data. This is achieved by the simple expedient of reformulating the problem focus after each round of information-gathering activity. To attain comparable facility in the multiple-problem context of INTERNIST-II will require the much more elaborate control strategies that characterize problem-solving methods of artificial intelligence.

REFERENCES

[1] Ledley, R. S., and L. B. Lusted. 1959. Reasoning foundation of medical diagnosis: Symbolic logic, probability and value theory and our understanding of how physicians reason. *Science* 130:9.

[2] Nordyke, J. F., C. A. Kulikowski, and C. W. Kulikowski, 1971. A comparison of methods for the automated diagnosis of thyroid dysfunction. *Comput. Biomed. Res.* 4:374–389.

[3] Patrick, E. A., F. P. Stelmack, and L. Y-L. Shen. 1974. Review of pattern recognition in medical diagnosis and consulting relative to a new system model. *IEEE Trans.*, SMC-4, no. 1:1–16.

[4] Ledley, R. S. 1969. Practical problems in the use of computers in medical diagnosis. *Proc. IEEE* 57:1900–1919.

[5] Feinstein, A. R. 1977. "The haze of Bayes, the aerial palaces of decision analysis, and the computerized Ouija board. *Clinical Biostatistics* 21:482–496.

[6] Szolovits, P., and S. G. Pauker. 1978. Categorical and probabilistic reasoning in medical diagnosis. *Artificial Intelligence* 11:115–144.

[7] Engle, R. L., B. J. Flehinger, and L. L. Leveridge. 1976. HEME: A computer aid to diagnosis of hematologic disease. *Bull. N.Y. Acad. Med.* 52:584–600.

[8] Ben-Bassat, M., and E. Lipnick. 1977. Diagnosis and treatment in MEDAS. *Proc. ACM,* 960–100.

[9] Wortman, P. M. 1972. Medical diagnosis: An information processing approach. *Comput. Biomed. Res.* 5:315–328.

[10] Patrick, E. A., and L. Y-L. Shen. 1975. *A systems approach to applying pattern recognition to medical diagnosis.* Purdue University Medical Computing Program, TR-EE 75–12.

[11] Warner, H. R., B. D. Rutherford, and B. Houtchens. 1972. A sequential Bayesian approach to history taking and diagnosis. *Comput. Biomed. Res.* 5:256–262.

[12] Gorry, G. A., and G. O. Barnett. 1968. Experience with a model of sequential diagnosis. *Comput. Biomed. Res.* 1:490–507.

[13] Bleich, H. L. 1972. Computer-based consultation: Electrolyte and acid-base disorders. *AJM* 53:285.

[14] Shortliffe, E. 1976. *Computer-based medical consultations: MYCIN*. New York: Elsevier.

[15] Weiss, S. M., C. A. Kulikowski, and A. Safir. 1977. A model-based consultation system for the long-term management of glaucoma. In *Proc. IJCAI-5, Cambridge, Mass.*, 826–832. Pittsburgh: Dept. of Computer Science, Carnegie-Mellon Univ.

[16] Silverman, H. 1975. *A digitalis therapy advisor, project MAC*. Mass. Inst. of Tech. Technical Report TR-143.

[17] Pauker, S. G., G. A. Gorry, J. P. Kassirer, and W. B. Schwartz. 1976. Toward the simulation of clinical cognition: Taking a present illness by computer. *AJM* 60:981–995.

[18] Pople, H. E., J. D. Myers, and R. A. Miller. 1975. The DIALOG model of diagnostic logic and its use in internal medicine. In *Proc. IJCAI-4, Tbilisi, USSR*. Cambridge, Mass.: Artificial Intelligence Laboratory, M.I.T.

[19] Pople, Harry E. 1977. The formation of composite hypotheses in diagnostic problem solving: An exercise in synthetic reasoning. In *Proc. IJCAI-5, Cambridge, Mass.* Pittsburgh: Dept. of Computer Science, Carnegie-Mellon Univ.

[20] Nilsson, N. J. 1971. *Problem solving methods in artificial intelligence*. San Francisco: McGraw-Hill.

[21] Winston, P. H. 1977. *Artificial intelligence*. Reading, Mass.: Addison-Wesley.

10

Diagnosis by Computer

Ernan McMullin

To what extent can the processes of clinical diagnosis be simulated by a computer program? In this paper I would like to look at INTERNIST-I, whose designers, J. D. Myers and H. E. Pople, made use of some interesting simulation techniques in constructing a program intended ultimately to cover the entire range of internal medicine.[1] It is certainly the most ambitious effort in this field so far; the Present Illness Program (PIP) of Pauker, Gorry, and Szolovits also employs a simulation approach to the clinical problems of internal medicine but is much more restricted in coverage.[2]

Programs of this kind are of particular interest to philosophers of science because they may be expected to illuminate the way in which one particularly complex form of scientific knowledge is arrived at. What is unique about INTERNIST-I is that it is aimed at replicating the diagnoses provided by a particular clinician, the distinguished internist Dr. Jack Myers. The criterion of success for this program is thus its ability to reach the same diagnostic outcome as Dr. Myers does in as wide a range of diagnostic problems as possible. The assumption is that if it could simulate the judgment of an expert, its aid could be relied on in guiding physicians engaged in the clinical process in internal medicine.

NONSIMULATION APPROACHES

Before turning to INTERNIST-I, it may be worth pointing out that a computer program intended to aid in clinical diagnosis need not be based on the simulation of the clinician's methods. Another quite different method is to accumulate a large amount of patient data and outcomes and then match the data on each new patient with those of the most closely matched subgroup in the record. The range of possible diagnoses can be derived by reference to this group. The method (which is sometimes called the "descriptive" or "regression" method) will work only in well-defined and limited areas of medicine where the classification of data presents no serious problems. Such a system is in operation at Duke Medical Center, for example, to handle coronary artery disease.[3] Systems like this one have two significant advantages: storage and analysis capacities that go far beyond those of a single clinician, and the possibility of accumulating new data in order to improve the diagnostic capability of the system.

A rather similar sort of system is often used by meteorologists for weather prediction. The computer stores as many potentially relevant data as possible, relevance being estimated by sophisticated statistical methods. The weather in a particular area can then be forecast by tracing what followed past weather configurations as nearly similar as possible to the present one. One need not know *why* the variables relate in the way they do, only *that* they do so in a reasonably stable manner. A system like this one can work very well to provide reliable predictions. And if prediction and explanation were *really* symmetrical with one another so that one could go directly from one to the other, as the logical positivists thought one could, a predictive system like this would simulate real science. But correlations of this sort are only the beginning of the scientific inquiry; they are not explanatory in their own right except in the very weakest sense.[4]

Computing systems of this matching kind are devised with the peculiar strengths of the computer in mind. One begins by asking what it does best. The simulation method, on the other hand, requires the computer to model the principles and procedures of the *clinician,* at least in certain aspects. Clinicians are already doing a good job of diagnosis. If we can simulate what they are doing, even approximately, we will have the equivalent of a second opinion available on-line when troublesome cases arise. That, at least, is the hope.

THE SIMULATION OF A SKILL

In a well-known book, Michael Polanyi underlined the fact that such skills as those of the clinician are mainly tacit. They are not learned from a manual, nor are they ever set out explicitly in the ordinary exercise of the skill.[5] To what extent can the computer scientist elicit the principles of their craft from clinicians? From the philosopher's point of view, this is one of the most fascinating aspects of the INTERNIST program. Dr. Myers writes: "I analyzed many cases for [Dr. Pople, the program designer]; he saw the principles involved, and that was the basis of INTERNIST-I." It was not, therefore, a matter of setting down principles formulated in advance. Rather, an outsider inferred them from the practice of the clinician, as well as from the clinician's answers to key questions. The program designer can attempt to formulate a principle that would account for some aspect of actual clinical practice. Or he can ask the clinician to try to make explicit the principles that guide him in making certain decisions. Dr. Myers remarks: "This resulted in much more introspection in regard to my own diagnostic processes and changed somewhat my own behavior as a physician." The computer scientist's questions forced him to try to clarify what it was he was doing, at the risk of getting it wrong. The principles thus arrived at introspectively would have the status of explanatory hypotheses. They would be tested by utilizing the computer program to make particular diagnostic moves and then testing these by seeing what the clinician would do in these cases.

The designer of such a computer program approaches the clinical process somewhat as a chemist, say, might approach a particular sort of chemical process in an effort to understand it by means of a hypothetical model. The links in the model must have some plausibility in their own right, but the model as a whole is tested by the inferences (predictions, instructions, diagnoses) it enables the scientist to draw. This is standard retroductive method.[6] What makes the simulation of the clinical process rather different, however, is first that the process is not at all a stable physical one, like the motion of a planet or the dissolving of a chemical. It is not the same from instance to instance; no two clinicians operate in precisely the same way or come up with the same diagnoses when circumstances repeat. Second, the clinical process is not an invariant; it is not at all the same today as it was a century ago. Third, the very effort to elucidate it (as Dr. Myers wryly notes) may well alter it. Since the process is a sociopsychological one, it might seem that a closer analogy could be drawn in the social sciences. Yet this analogy is not satisfactory either. To the extent that the clinical process is "scientific" (produces reliable knowledge in an explanatory context), it is governed in part by the norm of predictive success. And this gives it a degree of robustness that social processes ordinarily do not attain. It has to be reasonably effective in terms of such constraints as biopsy checks, postmortems, and of course therapy. Thus the principles governing it cannot be regarded simply as conventions, as the contingent product of a culture or of a particular subgroup. There is an external reference against which the skills, and the principles underlying them, must constantly be tested.

Is this the "chauvinism of Western scientific medicine" against which anthropologists, and philosophers like Paul Feyerabend, warn us?[7] There need be nothing chauvinistic about a reference to effective therapy, say, as a standard against which clinical practice has to be evaluated. But of course, this would not suffice to discriminate in favor of "scientific" medicine under all circumstances. Nor indeed should it. "Effective therapy" is a very broad qualification. Not only can folk medicine claim a considerable degree of therapeutic success in certain contexts, but the influence of suggestion is recognized (and utilized) within conventional "scientific" medicine itself. Further, it is often difficult to determine whether a particular therapy has been effective—that is, whether a cure has been accomplished, and if it has, whether this has really been due to the ministrations of the doctor.

Where the more explicitly scientific style of diagnosis scores is, of course, where there is a recognized pathology. The validity of the diagnosis can, in principle, be directly tested, even prior to therapy, in the case of infectious or parasitic diseases, cancer, heart disease, and the like. In such cases, medicine interlinks with biology, and a very broad network of empirical generalizations and explanatory models can be called on. On the other hand, where no pathological markers are known or where the causalities involved in therapy cannot be scrutinized, the scientific credentials of even the most therapeutically successful diagnosis are notoriously hard to establish.[8]

Critics have charged that the scientific aspect of the process of clinical diagnosis has been stressed too strongly in recent decades; diagnosis is not in the end (they urge) a purely scientific affair. We shall return to this issue, but first let us look more closely at the problem of simulating clinical diagnosis in one area of medicine where the "scientific" model seems to work fairly well.

THE CHOICE OF PROGRAM

The diagnostic problem is to infer from a set of manifestations (history, physical examination, tests) to a specific disorder or set of disorders.[9]

One or another of the manifestations might be pathognomonic, that is, might be linked uniquely with one disease only, in which case diagnosis is easy. But much more often this will not be so, and there will be more than one possible candidate. The clinician must try to assess the likelihood of these different possible explanations of the manifestations, and then go on, if possible, to suggest new types of manifestation to be explored in a progressive attempt to designate a single explanation as the "correct" one. There are thus two phases, the preliminary assessment of the most likely alternatives and the systematic ruling out of as many of these as possible.

There are several strategies a program might follow. Since it is attempting to determine likelihoods, the most obvious candidate might seem to be a scheme of Bayesian probabilities, using relative frequencies of disease and manifestation in a specified population.[10] Unfortunately, this does not work very well. The main reason is that the manifestations are not independent of one another but may be causally linked in intricate ways. In a Bayesian scheme, each of these would be regarded as a separate index, affecting probability in its own right. A further difficulty, one that often arises in practical applications of the elegant Bayesian formalism, is that prior probabilities are very difficult to estimate in the clinical context. What should the reference population be? How restricted a class ought one consider? The prior probability of uterine cancer will obviously depend on the sex, the age, the history, of the patient.

A quite different strategy would be to look for *patterns* of manifestations that are characteristic of particular disorders. This combinatorial approach is frequently utilized by the clinician. But it is difficult to make it into an effective program since the link between disease and manifestation is often a loose one. So many variants on the pattern have to be recognized that the problems of program design are formidable. Yet, as Clouser and Suppes point out, proper simulation will obviously have to work not just with manifestations taken singly but with *clusters,* where each cluster is characteristic of a disorder, yet is relatively loosely defined. This would give some kind of "bonus" for linkage, especially causal linkage, of manifestations into a single pattern.

The new program, INTERNIST-II (recently, for legal reasons, renamed CADUCEUS) is designed to meet this challenge.[11] It looks for pattern, rather than simply summing over the individual relations of manifestation to diagnostic hypothesis, as INTERNIST-I does. The program is still in the planning stages, and compared with

INTERNIST-I will be far more difficult to carry through to the operational level of attaching weights to alternative diagnostic hypotheses. It is quite unlike the earlier program in its general construction. It is built around two types of diagram combined in a complex way to order the space of possible hypotheses. One type of diagram is *causal;* it displays the causal relations of manifestation and disorder insofar as these are known. The other presents a *nosology,* a hierarchical structure of disease categories, based on some principle of ordering (e.g., by the organ affected).

Where it is possible to carry through a clinical diagnosis by means of a fully causal diagram, the goals of theoretical science have been satisfied, and the patient's symptoms have been explained in the conventional "scientific" way. But this is rarely possible, in the initial diagnostic stages especially, where information is ordinarily quite incomplete. To rely on a purely causal diagnostic approach would enormously increase the search space, beyond even the abundant capacities of computers. That is why "constrictors" are introduced from a chosen nosology. The aim of clinical diagnosis is not, in any event, to achieve a fully scientific understanding of the patient's ailment. The aim is effective therapy, and for this a causal account is often not needed. The clinician can do quite well with a lesser degree of understanding, although when anomalous results appear, it is obviously a help to know what the causal links are.

My concern here, however, is not with INTERNIST-II (CADUCEUS) but with the older program, which depended on a quasi-Bayesian approach, estimating the contribution to the diagnostic picture of each clinical manifestation separately. The hope was that enough redundancy could be built into the system to overcome its obvious inability to simulate the "patterning" capacity of the good clinician.

INTERNIST-I

INTERNIST-I relates individual manifestations (M) to postulated explanatory disorders (D) by means of three numbers, the combination of which gives the epistemic "weight" of each D-hypothesis. The choice of these three factors is motivated by the simulation aim of the program. It is believed that working clinicians intuitively rely on "something like" these factors. Furthermore, the "strength" of two of the three factors is estimated in each case by asking the clinician what his "informed guess" would be, thus once again relying on simulation.

The most important of the three numbers is "evoking strength" (ES), relating manifestation (M) to disorder (D). It is the likelihood of D, given M. L(D,M) is estimated subjectively by the clinician on an integer scale running from 5 (high) to 0 (low). The clinician asks himself, "When I encounter M, how seriously should I entertain the hypothesis of D?" Such a question is clearly context-dependent. ES should depend first of all on the frequency of D in the population to which the patient belongs. Clouser puts it this way: "The strength of a physician's initial disposition to regard his patient as having a certain illness is directly proportional to the incidence of that disease in the population he serves." This way of putting it is rather too Bayesian, perhaps, but the claim that ES must be affected by the actual frequency of occurrence of D in the population seems fair enough. ES should depend, second, on the likelihood that D and M are causally related. Clouser would prefer to restrict the analysis to empirical frequencies (in this case, the frequency with which D is associated with M in the target population): "We need not be concerned with causal relationships, but only with sheer correlations." Myers on the other hand prefers to build a specifically causal emphasis into ES. Finally, ES should depend on the availability of alternatives to D as causal explanations of M. The strength with which M evokes D will depend on whether M could be brought about by other causes $D_1, D_2 \ldots$, as well as on how commonly these other causes occur. Myers calls this "specificity." D might be common in the population, it might invariably bring about M, but M would still not evoke D very strongly if M were also brought about by a number of other common diseases.

Analyzed in this way, ES suggests the Bayesian calculation for P(D,M), that is, the probability of D, given M. But evoking strength in the INTERNIST-I program is deliberately not expressed in terms of probabilities, frequencies, or specific populations. Nor is it explicitly broken down into three subfactors. It is a single subjective likelihood estimate on a conventional scale. The reconstruction given above of the factors that *should* influence it is a tentative one, since Dr. Myers has little to say about how he arrives at his ES numbers, about which clues he relies on, and how he weights these relatively to one another.

Clouser gives us an important reminder that the "manifestations" here are not the neat items they are in ordinary probability calculations. A laboratory result may be on the borderline between a "positive" and a "negative." A laboratory specimen may be untypical. The clinician who takes the history may not use quite the right category for a finding or may overlook something important. Clouser believes that these sorts of ambiguities and contingencies can be allowed for by statistical methods and sees this as one of the advantages of the computer. But obviously, building these kinds of margin into an actual system could be next to impossible in many cases.

ES works as verification. And an ES measure amalgamated over all supporting data can be used in a preliminary way as a "constrictor," to reduce the range of broad generic alternatives the program should first investigate. But what if there are manifestations one would expect to accompany D and they are not found? Ought not this to refute the hypothesis? In clinical medicine, as elsewhere in science, strict falsificationism would be naive. But what weight is to be given to anomalies of this kind? INTERNIST-I here uses a second measure, the *frequency number* (FN), again ranging from 5 (all) to 0 (none), which measures the frequency in the target population with which D is accompanied by M. If the FN is high, then the anomaly of a missing M is serious. The FN measure is used, therefore, to estimate the weight of counterevidence. It is based not on a clinician's estimate of likelihood (as ES is) but on empirical frequency counts in medical records.

This is an interesting decision on the part of the program designers. On the face of it, it might seem that ES too might just as easily be derived from medical records, thus eliminating the need for a "subjective" estimate on the part of a clinician. But this would be to remove one of the main simulation features of the program, and one upon which its sensitivity as an "evoker" of hypotheses so largely depends.

Ought a strong anomaly to eliminate a particular D from consideration? Does it, in actual clinical practice, do so? The extensive critical discussion of Popper's falsificationist theory of science would remind us that several other alternatives are usually worth exploring in such cases. The most obvious one is that a mistake has been made: scrutinize the anomalous manifestation for error. In clinical medicine, this is an ever-present possibility: unrepresentative laboratory results, concealment or forgetfulness on the part of the patient, effects of an earlier unnoted disease . . . Or it may be that the description of D can be refined in such a way as to give a new FN for the offending manifestation. The INTERNIST-I program does not attempt to deal with these alternatives, but the alert clinician would have them in mind where the intuitive evoking strength of a particular D is high and the intuitive weight of an anomalous M is equally high. This is one of the contexts in which the user of the program would be helped by having a display available showing how the particular recommendation of the program has been arrived at.

So now we have two measures, one positive (ES) and one negative (FN). How are these to be combined into a single measure of likelihood? Probability theory provides no answer. Recent debates between the defenders of verificationist and falsificationist theories of science suggest that an answer is unlikely to be forthcoming from philosophers either. Can one have any assurance that there *is* a mathematical weighting function that would give the "correct" answer in all cases? Not so far as I can see. No intuitive principle tells us what to do with an ES of 5 and a contrary FN of 3. What the designers of INTERNIST-I did was to begin from an initially plausible joint weighting factor and then adjust it in order to achieve best reults in a range of specific clinical cases.[12] "Best results" here means, of course, best fit with Dr. Myers's own recommendations in these same cases. This might suggest a continued process of fine-tuning, but in point of fact the designers have as yet modified the weighting factor only once, and it remains a very crude measure of the relative weight to be given the different types of number. The assumption that there *is* such a weighting factor that remains mathematically stable over all contexts is, of course, open to question, but without such an assumption the program could not be constructed.

So far we have encountered two logically different sorts of manifestation, those that are accounted for by a particular D-hypothesis and those that count against such a hypothesis. But many of the manifestations will not fall in either of these categories; they will be neutral in regard to D.[13] D neither accounts for them nor is challenged by them.[14] What ought one do about this "residue" when assessing the value of a particular D-hypothesis? Myers's answer is to assign an "*import* number" (IN) to weigh the clinical importance of each M, taken as a separate clinical indication. (Note that IN, unlike ES and FN, is attached to M's singly, not to (M,D) pairs.) Myers asks himself, "How readily can this M be disregarded?" This then allows him to estimate the total "weight" of the manifestations that are not taken into account in proposing a particular D-hypothesis.

Ought such a measure to count *against* this D? This is, in fact, the way in which IN is taken in the system. But it seems very odd. After all, a second co-occurrent disease may very well explain the residue of manifestations left untouched by the original D-hypothesis. So the fact that D does not account for that group of manifestations ought not, logically speaking, to count against the first D-hypothesis.

IN could, of course, serve to estimate the "importance" of the undiagnosed residue, after a particular diagnosis has been made, "im-

portance" in the sense of how important, clinically speaking, it is not
to terminate the diagnosis at that point. But IN, taken in this way,
ought not (it would seem) to count *against* the original D-hypothesis.
Part of the problem lies in the ambiguity of the term *import*. Dr. Myers
asks, "How important is this M in diagnosis?" This could mean
"important in leading to a correct diagnosis" or "medically serious so
that it must be accounted for." (The term *disregard,* also used by
Dr. Myers, exhibits the same ambiguity between an epistemic and a
practical sense.) These two sorts of "import" would obviously interact
with the other two measures in rather different ways. In his intuitive
assignment of IN measures, Dr. Myers appears to have had both senses
of *import* in mind, so that the import numbers are a sort of amalgamated
measure.[15]

It does not seem that IN ought to be given much, if any, epistemic
weight. The epistemic import of an anomaly is already supplied by
the relevant FN. And the epistemic import of an M that fails to support
a D-candidate is captured already by the correspondingly low ES
measure. Nothing more is needed. The "residue" list (low ES, low
FN, in relation to this D) is simply not relevant to the assessment of
the likelihood of the D-candidate. Of course, if there are M's in the
residue list with a high IN in the sense of, say, life-threatening
symptoms, the clinician will want to press on to find a second conjoint
hypothesis, an additional D, to account for them.

If the IN numbers are used to quantify the residue list relative to a
particular D and this measure then is used negatively to diminish the
likelihood of D, this will bias the program in favor of the more global
explanatory hypotheses. It might be said that here again the program
simulates the real clinician who is quite likely to prefer a single
diagnostic hypothesis that leaves as few high-import manifestations
unexplained as possible. It might also be argued that a *single* explanatory hypothesis is clinically more likely than a string of D-candidates
that causally are relatively independent of one another. But it could
be argued on the other side that the more global hypothesis is already
sufficiently recognized by its high ES measure. And after all, a multiplicity of unrelated or barely related disorders *is* quite often the correct
diagnosis.

The import number is, perhaps, the feature of INTERNIST-I which
is farthest removed from the Bayesian scheme. It would have no
analogue in the natural sciences. It is interesting that Myers and Pople
found it necessary to introduce this conceptually troublesome measure

in their efforts to simulate a clinician's reasoning. On the face of it, it would seem that laying heavy negative weight on IN could lead the clinician away from the correct explanatory hypothesis, the hypothesis on which the best therapeutic advice could be based. So much, then, for the first round of assessment carried out by INTERNIST-I.

PURSUING A DIAGNOSIS

At this point a fourth class of M's becomes crucial. This consists of the manifestations one would *expect* to accompany a particular D-hypothesis but which remain as yet untested. The second use of the computer program is to suggest which tests should be made and in what order. In principle, one would want to begin with the M's that have a high FN measure for the D's that are the strongest candidates. But this may mean using dangerous tests unnecessarily soon. So INTERNIST-I for the second time (the first was with IN) introduces nonepistemic values. The different test procedures are divided into three levels on the basis of risk, expense, and discomfort to the patient. Level 0 contains the routine general tests; level 1 contains nonroutine tests that are not expensive, risky, or invasive; level 2 contains the remainder, and in principle, these could have an internal ranking in terms of the three types of negative value mentioned, amalgamated in some agreed way. Tests from the last two levels are called up only when necessary in the final stages of the differential diagnosis.

As the test results come in, each D-candidate will either gain in strength or diminish to the point of being ruled out. That is the hope, at least. If at this point there are still several strong contenders (strong in terms of their combined ES/FN/IN measure), the *Discriminate* segment of the program goes into operation. This corresponds very roughly to the notion of "crucial experiment," since the aim is to choose tests that will discriminate between the remaining candidates by supporting some (if possible, one) using the ES measure and tending to rule out the others by the FN measure.

The program assigns a quantitative measure to each D-candidate, and the aim is to raise this measure for one of the candidates to as high a level as possible while reducing the measure on all other candidates to the point that, by comparison, they may effectively be disregarded. In the final *Pursue* mode of the program, the leading candidate is investigated in detail. This is done by checking in the fourth M-class (manifestations not yet investigated) for those M's which would have the highest ES measure for this particular D-candidate. It is assumed that all those M's with a high FN measure for this D-candidate would already have been evaluated by the program in the earlier modes. Such a measure is not a *sufficient* condition for a high ES measure, as we have seen, although it is a component in it. Thus, a different class of M's would be called on by looking for those with a high ES measure, even though those with a high FN measure for this D (those which are ordinarily associated with this D) would be likely to form a considerable part of those with high ES measure for D.

The *Pursue* mode is continued until one of the candidates is separated from its nearest competitor by the margin that the program has been set to recognize as "satisfactory" or until the clinician decides to terminate it short of that. He might do this because the tests needed for further discrimination are unacceptable or because even with all available tests given, no single hypothesis yet emerges sufficiently far ahead of the others. There are, after all, situations where the clinician is unable to come up with a single reasonably firm diagnosis; since the program simulates a clinician, it will not always be able to conclude. Of course, the clinician might be able at this point to come up with a novel suggestion, a different strategy, or the like, one that can intuitively be assessed as having some chance of success. INTERNIST-I cannot do this.

Nor can it accumulate data from past trials to correct and sharpen the individual measures and the relative weightings built into it. This would require a very complicated additional level in the program. Dr. Myers can update the measures, basing his judgment on the medical literature and on his clinical experience. But there is no automatic learning function built into INTERNIST-I as there is, for example, in the Duke coronary-artery program already mentioned.

When a particular D can be proposed as the best clinical solution for a subset of the M's, the program then is set to turn to the remaining M's (*Recycle* mode) and run through the process again, especially (one supposes) if there are some high IN measures among the unexplained M's. A fourth measure is now used in addition to the three we have already seen: this is the "link" (L) value that is assigned to D's that are in any way causally related to the D that has already been diagnosed. The assumption is that the presence of D heightens the likelihood of other disorders also, and these ought therefore to be assigned a "bonus" in the next round of assessment. The L measure is generated from the ES and FN relations between the two D's. It could in principle be based on the evidence of frequency counts only, but Dr. Myers seems to lay more weight on the determination of properly causal relationships.

The fact that when the diagnosis has reached a particular disorder, there may well be other disorders still to be discovered, recalls once again one of the most troublesome features of this entire simulation project. In the natural sciences and in medical research also, one tries to isolate single problems. One focuses on a single issue at a time as far as possible. In clinical medicine, one cannot do this. The individual patient sets the problem. And it may be a causally complex one, either in the sense of a causally unrelated set of disorders, or what is worse, a causally related set where the causal interactions alter the manifestations in barely predictable ways. The various M and D relationships may alter if another D comes in to complicate the picture.

The first problem that this sets for the programmer (or for that matter, the clinician) is that of *partitioning,* as Dr. Myers calls it. Let us go back to the beginning. There may be a hundred or more manifestations to cope with. Obviously, these can be partitioned in different ways. And each partitioning could suggest a different set of (related or unrelated) disorders that could be responsible for the set of manifestations, taken as a whole. Thus the choice of *initial* partitioning could well determine the outcome.[16] Ought one to favor an initial hypothesis that explains the largest possible number of M's in terms of a single disorder? This is the principle that problem solving in other areas would tend to follow, since unexplained data would ordinarily count *against* the hypothesis proposed. But in the clinical case one is allowed to set up an independent noncompeting explanation (or set of explanations) for the other data. This means (as we have already seen in discussing the IN measure above) that unexplained data ought not really to be counted against the first hypothesis, unless one has exhausted the possible explanations of the residue and come up with nothing satisfactory. But the combination possibilities are so enormous here that this kind of assurance could probably not be arrived at in situations of even moderate complexity.

What would, in principle, be best would be simultaneous consideration of all the possible partitionings of the M's that would give rise to different sets of alternatives, and then a decision as to which set had the highest likelihood measure. But this sort of "parallel" processing is barely reachable at the present stage of programming because of the immense number of alternatives that would have to be run through. It would be even more difficult in parallel mode to know what recommendations to make in regard to "unexplored" M's, tests to be made, questions to be asked, and so on.

Thus, INTERNIST-I follows a "serial" or "sequential" procedure, taking one range of M's at a time and concluding with this set, more or less, before asking what quality of explanation is available for the residue. This is, as Pople and Simon remind us, the strategy followed by human clinicians, so far as one can tell, so that from the simulation standpoint this is the correct strategy to follow. But ideally, it seems clear that a simultaneous consideration of all the partitionings and their submeasures would be more likely to yield the correct diagnosis. Serial consideration is likely to skew the process, at least to some extent, by focusing on one range of the data to the relative exclusion of the rest.

The partitioning used in INTERNIST-I depends, Dr. Myers tells us, on *homology;* "where two or more disease models are homologous, they are competitors, but if they are not, they are considered as possibly both being present." How the homology estimate is constructed within the system is not quite clear. One possibility would be a function based on the FN measure, in terms of which one could antecedently determine the "closeness" of any two D's by how many M's they have in common, perhaps quantified by the respective FN measures. And the program could then determine in the first screening of alternatives whether more or less unrelated alternatives are being considered for different ranges of the data.

Another approach, coming from the M rather than the D side, would be to make the separation threshold between any two M's depend on the frequency with which they are found as part of the same diagnostic complex. And then the initial manifestation list could be tested for clusters of related M's. There would then be a question as to how the homologies, so specified, would be used to establish the "best" partitioning. But what INTERNIST-I *actually* does (so far as I can see) is to focus on the M-list associated with the D-candidate of broadest scope and highest composite likelihood in order to establish the division between the "Considering" and "Disregarding" lists in the *Rule-out* and *Discriminate* phases of the operation. But this is obviously problematic since the top alternatives will not have the same M-lists, so that to set a particular M under "Considering" instead of "Disregarding" may bias the measure toward one alternative and away from another.

SHORTCOMINGS

I have already noted some of the shortcomings of INTERNIST-I. In their papers, Pople and Myers mention some others. But they stress that for well over one-half of the disease entities of internal medicine, the system gives quite good results, not quite up to those of a good clinician, but better on the average than those of doctors under the level of clinician. Still, the deficiencies of INTERNIST-I have seemed sufficiently serious to warrant, as we have seen, the construction of a new system, INTERNIST-II (CADUCEUS), which, in principle at least, should be able to overcome some of the principal defects of the earlier system.

The main problem with INTERNIST-I, as we have seen, is its inability to simulate the clinician's patterning ability, the ability to recognize common M-clusters *as* clusters of a causally related sort. The clinician does not consider each M separately and assign a weight to it implicitly; the real clinical process is not even approximately Bayesian (as INTERNIST-I is). Allied with this is the partitioning difficulty, only partially met in INTERNIST-I, not only the initial formulation of the diagnostic problem but the continued focus of the program on one set of M's rather than another. How is a "focus" to be constructed? INTERNIST-II introduces a double structure, causal and taxonomic, in an effort to provide the requisite search pattern.

One further associated shortcoming in the earlier program is the fact that it operates *serially*, considering only one problem-focus at a time and modifying it as new information comes in. The danger here is, of course, that it may go off in the wrong direction and follow a blind alley, neglecting other possible formulations of the problem. What is needed here is a *parallel* processing of many alternative structurings of the diagnostic problem at each stage. This needs, as we have seen, an enormously larger computer power, since the search space is so great.

Another inadequacy in INTERNIST-I is its inability to register the developmental aspect of diseases, the way they present over time. To the clinician, the way in which a disorder develops, the sequence in which the manifestations appear and the intervals between them, can be very significant. Here, too, what the clinician picks out is the characteristic pattern rather than just the single items. To take account of this, the program not only would need to add a temporal qualifier to the M's but would need a further clustering function where the significance of an M would be affected by its temporal relationship with other M's. This too would require a large increase in computer power.

A number of conceptual difficulties were already mentioned. The IN measure seems somewhat ambiguous both in concept and in use. The degree of dependence of the ES and the FN measures on the population to which the patient belongs can cause serious difficulty, especially since this population cannot be defined in a unique way. The relative weighting assigned by the system-designers to the three measures in computing an overall likelihood value of a particular D-candidate is very hard to evaluate. Despite these shortcomings, however, it must be said that the preliminary dissection of the various elements of diagnostic judgment made by the designers of INTER-NIST-I already illuminates the epistemic structure of this kind of judgment in a helpful way.

TWO SENSES OF *DIAGNOSIS*

Our examination of INTERNIST-I has helped us grasp some of the logical structures that underlie the act of clinical diagnosis. How far can the analogy be pushed between diagnosis and scientific explanation? To what extent ought we to expect the procedures of INTERNIST to reflect the procedures of theoretical natural science? For example, is the primary aim of clinical diagnosis to find out the nature of the disease entity involved? What, in short, are the criteria for success in a clinical diagnosis?

In a recent essay, Caroline Whitbeck is critical of the tendency on the part of the designers of INTERNIST-I to adopt the "diagnostic model" of clinical reasoning, a model that would make diagnostic specificity the main goal of the clinician and would (mistakenly, in her view) define diagnosis as "the determination of the nature of the disease":[17]

> Although this computer program seems useful for the purpose for which it was designed, to act as a consultant to other internists, its single-minded devotion to the rapid attainment of diagnostic precision disregards the danger of harming the patient in the process. Thus we will be misled if we take it to be a heuristic that represents a prototype of problem-solving in internal medicine.[18]

In short, her complaint about the program is that "its single-minded pursuit of diagnostic specificity departs from the standards of good clinical reasoning."

How might Pople and Myers respond to this? I suspect that they would be quite happy to settle for the admission that the system is useful for the purpose for which it was designed. They might go on to note that the use of INTERNIST-I as a teaching tool for clinicians-to-be would have its dangers if the teacher were to forget that it is an idealized model, a first approximation from which many important features of the clinician's activities have been omitted. They would, perhaps, add that it is not too likely that this *would* be forgotten by a competent clinical teacher. Still, they might admit that the intellectual challenge represented by the problem-solving side of the clinical task could perhaps be so heightened by the INTERNIST "game" that the values associated with patient well-being might be insufficiently realized by some. One would not, after all, want an apprentice clinician to spend all of his or her time glued to the console, working on clinical problems from the NEJM!

But is it the case that INTERNIST *is* governed always by epistemic principles and that broader clinical values are laid aside?[19] We have seen that in two respects it does recognize these values: in its ordering of tests according to danger, expense, and discomfort, and in its (somewhat ambiguous) use of the import number. The program attempts to progress as far as possible with the more easily obtained information first. And the requests for further information are evaluated by the clinician in any event. The clinician is not expected to authorize every information request; in the actual operation of the program, as sample readouts show, the frequent response "GO" from the clinician ("the information requested will not, as yet at least, be sought") throws the initiative back to the program to find a different question.

Dr. Myers appears to suggest a third way in which nonepistemic values affect program outcome. In discussing the principles of diagnostic practice, he notes that a good clinician will investigate the more life-threatening possibilities first; he or she will also give prior attention to disorders for which effective therapy is available. He quotes Dr. Levine approvingly: "I do not care whether I make a diagnosis of multiple sclerosis; there is little I can do about it anyway. I want to make sure that this patient does not have a tumor of the spinal cord which can be removed surgically and cure the patient."[20]

The reader might easily be led to infer that these two further value orderings have been incorporated into INTERNIST. In fact they have not. Here, then, are two dimensions of clinical practice that have had to be laid aside in this first effort at simulation. To incorporate them would not be impossible, but it would add two more levels of complexity to the already formidable task of the program designer. One device that might help would be to enable the clinician to instruct the program to focus on any of the listed alternatives that seem to him or her especially life-threatening, in order to rule them out, if possible, before investigating anything else. Or the clinician could instruct the program to disregard temporarily an alternative for which no therapy is available.

INTERNIST-I, in short, could do more. And it could be misused by someone who thought it did everything. At this rather banal level everyone would surely agree. Further, there would be general agreement that the clinician's primary aim must be to help the patient and that identifying the disease must rank as secondary to this. The ultimate criterion of clinical success is that diagnosis should lead to effective therapy, not that it should provide an understanding of what the disorder is.

Where disagreement occurs is in regard to the proper usage of the term *diagnosis*. Ought we to take diagnosis to be the properly *epistemic* part of clinical reasoning? Value constraints (risk, cost, etc.) would then be extraneous to it. They would pertain to the structure of clinical reasoning, of course, not to the logic of *diagnosis*, strictly speaking. Ordinary usage seems to favor this: "From the symptoms and the biopsy, I can diagnose with complete confidence that a tumor is responsible. But I fear that no therapy is going to be of any use." This would count (I think) as a successful diagnosis, even though the overriding therapeutic aims of the clinical enterprise have not been realized. "He diagnosed the malady but killed the patient in doing it." A correct diagnosis but bad clinical reasoning. "It is inappropriate to seek to discover whether a patient's condition is operable or not if the patient is unable to survive an operation." The inappropriateness here would usually be termed "clinical" rather than "diagnostic."[21]

On the other hand, one could take *diagnosis* to refer to the entire activity engaged in by the clinician at the investigative stage. It will then have both epistemic and nonepistemic aspects. The clinician seeks to know the causes only insofar as this aids the patient's restoration to health. If the patient is unnecessarily endangered by what the clinician does, this is bad diagnostic practice. "Doing X for the sake of Y" blends two sets of norms, and can therefore fail on two separate sorts of grounds. (Can it be said to succeed if Y is not in fact achieved, just so long as the doing of X did not itself threaten Y?)

The issue here can become analytically quite intricate. It may suffice to sum up in irenic fashion by allowing that either usage is possible. Each has its advantage and its disadvantages. The narrower usage seems closer to the traditional sense of the term *to diagnose,* whereas the broader one reflects the complexity of the norms governing the investigative task of the clinician.

One point, however, is clear. What INTERNIST-I seeks to simulate is this broader activity. The simulation is only partial, of course, as simulation always is. Since the aim of the designers is to produce a program that would help the clinician somewhat as a consultant might, it would be even better if they could successfully simulate the *total* investigative activity of the clinician, working under the same constraints and value norms, if possible, as a clinician would. These latter are much harder to simulate than epistemic principles would be, in part because of their variability from one clinician to another and in part because of the extreme difficulty, noted above, in deciding upon a relative weighting between epistemic and nonepistemic ordering principles.

The INTERNIST-I program is thus broader in scope than "diagnosis" (in its purely epistemic sense) that abstracts from clinical activity only those aspects which bear on the scientific determination of the disorders that are at the source of the manifestations presented. If one uses the term in this narrower sense, then one would have to say INTERNIST-I makes at least some attempt to go beyond the strictly "diagnostic" aspects of clinical reasoning in its simulation aims. If, however, the term is used in the broader sense, then INTERNIST-I can be simply described as simulating "diagnosis," even if very incompletely. If this distinction is observed, a lot of needless argument can be avoided.

DIAGNOSIS AS SCIENTIFIC EXPLANATION

At the beginning of this essay, I noted that INTERNIST-I is of interest to philosophers of science because of its attempt to simulate what clinicians do when they set about determining what the causes are in specific clinical cases. The differences between what they are doing and what physicists or medical researchers do have been made plain along the way. Does INTERNIST-I—or for that matter, clinical diagnosis itself—have much to offer the philosopher, therefore, who seeks to understand better what science is like?

The natural sciences follow a "Galilean" method of idealization and experiment. They break down the complicated happenings of the familiar world into their single factors by setting up artificial experimental contexts where the influence of all agencies except those explicitly under consideration is eliminated or at least controlled. The possible disadvantage here is *distortion*. One may be creating an artifact that will not really illuminate the behavior of the complex entities of the everyday world. The behavior of an animal in laboratory surroundings may not always be a good index of what it will do in its natural state. Nevertheless, Galilean science does allow us to formulate a theoretical understanding of the web of agencies that make up our "natural" world.

Clinical medicine, as we have seen, does not aim at theoretical understanding. It aims at the practical goal of therapy, though it uses whatever theoretical science is available. Second, it deals primarily with the individual, not with the class. Insofar as it does attempt to understand a situation, it is the situation of an individual organism, with all the contingencies of history ineradicably present in its structure and activity.[22] The test of success in a diagnosis is not the formulation of a generalization or a theory but the understanding of what is "wrong" in this particular case.

The engineer and the architect, likewise, deal with individuals. Their problems arise from concrete contingent situations that cannot be artificially simplified to make their task easier. The road has to go through this particular piece of terrain; the architect has to make the best of this piece of land. They too make use of whatever theoretical science is available to help them understand the complex practical problems with which they are faced.

The hero of *Zen and the Art of Motorcycle Maintenance* proposed the problem-solving of the motorcycle mechanic as an analogy for science generally.[23] This leads him into such a disastrously wrong assessment of science that it contributes to the psychological breakdown he ultimately experiences. The problem-solving situation of the mechanic is not, for many reasons, a particularly good analogy for that of the scientist. But because his work is partly diagnostic in character, it does bear some resemblance to that of the clinician. There are, however, several important differences. The operations of the engine are fully understood; there is no need for continuing research to understand its workings. Also the engine can be manipulated in any way one wishes; it can be broken down into its constituent parts for testing. The problem situation of the clinician, because of the likely presence in the patient of causalities that are not fully understood, is much closer to that of the research scientist.

History is another discipline where one must leave the complexities of the historical individual in place, as the clinician does, and try to understand them in all their contingency. Historians do not have the resources the clinician possesses to pursue a line of questioning and systematically test their hypotheses against the answers they receive. But they can make use of the resources of the social and psychological sciences, and they are held to norms of evidence that allow their claims to be tested. In both these respects their work has affinities with that of the social scientist. Where it differs is in its focus on the individual instead of the general.

"Science" is no single thing. It has many strands, and they interweave in odd ways. Clinical medicine is a particularly challenging knot in this web. It has affinities with natural science, with social science, with history, with art, even with motorcycle maintenance. But in the end it is a knot unlike any other. The challenge facing those who would simulate it is to untangle the many strands. Drs. Myers and Pople, and the many others now engaged in this task, ought to be the envy of philosophers who have been engaged in their own way in this sort of untangling for a long time.

NOTES

1. This essay began as a comment on the papers by J. D. Myers and K. D. Clouser at the Pittsburgh conference on which this volume is based. A first version of it appeared as "Diagnosis by Computer" in *The Journal of Medicine and Philosophy* 8 (1983): 5–27. (This special issue of the JMP was wrongly titled "Ethical Issues in Computer Diagnosis." "Ethical" was a printer's slip; it should have read "Conceptual.") In revising this earlier version I benefited from the comments of Bill Clancy and Ken Schaffner; for his patient answers to my constantly reformulated questions I am indebted to Harry Pople.

2. S. G. Pauker et al., "Towards the Simulation of Clinical Cognition: Taking a Present Illness by Computer," *American Journal of Medicine* 60

(1976): 981–995; P. Szolovits and S. G. Pauker, "Research on a Medical Consultation System for Taking the Present Illness," *Proceedings of the Third Illinois Conference on Medical Information Systems* (Chicago: University of Illinois at Chicago Circle, 1976), 299–320. For some useful comparisons between Pittsburgh's INTERNIST-I and the MIT/TUFTS PIP, see P. Szolovits and S. G. Pauker, "Categorical and Probabilistic Reasoning in Medical Diagnosis," *Artificial Intelligence* 11 (1978): 115–144.

3. R. A. Rosati, A. G. Wallace, and E. A. Stead, "The Way of the Future," *Archives of Internal Medicine* 131 (1973): 285–287. See also H. M. Schoolman and L. M. Bernstein, "Computer Use in Diagnosis, Prognosis and Therapy," *Science* 200 (1978): 926–931.

4. See E. McMullin, "Structural Explanation," *American Philosophical Quarterly* 15 (1978): 139–147.

5. M. Polanyi, *Personal Knowledge* (London: Routledge, 1958).

6. E. McMullin, "A Clinician's Quest for Certainty," in *Clinical Judgment: A Critical Appraisal,* ed. T. Engelhardt et al. (Dordrecht: Reidel), 115–129. See sec. 5, "Ampliative Inference."

7. P. Feyerabend, *Science in a Free Society* (London: New Left Bookstore, 1978). See part 2, sec. 9, "Nor Is Science Preferable because of Its Results."

8. See, e.g., A. Grunbaum, "Epistemological Liabilities of the Clinical Appraisal of Psychoanalytic Theory," *Nous* 14 (1980): 107–185.

9. Terms like *manifestation, disorder, disease,* raise difficult philosophical issues. But we shall have to leave these aside here.

10. P. Suppes, "The Logic of Clinical Judgment: Bayesian and Other Approaches," in *Clinical Judgment,* ed. Engelhardt et al., 145–159.

11. See H. Pople, "Heuristic Methods for Imposing Structure on Ill-structured Problems: The Structuring of Medical Diagnostics," in *Artificial Intelligence in Medicine,* ed. P. Szolovits (Boulder, Colo.: Westview Press, 1982), 119–190.

12. Myers and Pople do not discuss this in their published papers. K. Schaffner, however, provides a table of the numerical values associated with each of the ES, FN, and IN measures in a recent helpful review of INTERNIST-I ("Modeling Medical Diagnosis," *Synthèse* 47[1981]: 163–199). Thus, for example, an ES score of 5 is given 40, IN-5 gets 30. The summation of scores within each type is nonlinear; thus, two FN-3's sum as an FN-4, and two FN-4's sum as an FN-5. (This summation rule, once again, is based on the intuitive assessment of Dr. Myers.) The summed FN and IN values are subtracted from the summed ES values to give the weight of the proposed D-hypothesis relative to a particular set of M's.

13. For an M to be "neutral" it must have a low ES *and* a low FN with regard to the particular D-hypothesis. M_1 is accounted for by D_1 if M_1 is

usually associated with D_1, even though D_1 is rarely associated with M_1; M_1 would also be accounted for by D_1, if D_1 is usually associated with M_1, even though M_1 is rarely associated with D_1.

14. M may be said to *challenge* a particular D-hypothesis, when D would lead one to expect something *other* than this M. (*Manifestation* has to be taken broadly; it could be a *normal* blood-sugar reading, for instance.) In such a case, not-M would have a high FN in regard to this D.

15. Commentaries on INTERNIST-I reflect this same ambiguity. "Counting against a model are data expected but found negative, which are weighted in proportion to their frequency numbers in the considered disease and also in proportion to their import" (Pople, "Heuristic Methods," 179). If IN were actually used in this way to qualify the FN measures in order to compute the negative weight of the anomaly list, the sense of *import* would be the epistemic one: "How significant an anomaly would it be if this M were missing in the context of this D?" But surely this is already covered by the FN measure? Myers appears to say that *only* the FN measure is used to calculate the weight of the anomaly list. Caroline Whitbeck also appears to interpret IN epistemically. When she criticizes what she takes to be the lack of emphasis on properly clinical values in INTERNIST-I, she says that this "is illustrated by the lack of connection between the value labelled 'import' . . . and the actual hazard that the sign or symptom poses to the patient's well-being. What is called the 'import' of a sign in INTERNIST is only an indication of its diagnostic task" ("What Is Diagnosis? A Preface to the Investigation of Clinical Reasoning," *Metamedicine* [1981]: 319–329). Schoolman and Bernstein have yet another understanding of IN ("Computer Use," 929). They think that IN is used on the *positive* side to estimate the import of the M's that *are* explained by the D-candidate. This would not be at all equivalent to taking the combined IN measure of the "residue list" (a different set of M's) as a negative measure. One could, of course, take both, but it would seem to run contrary to Dr. Myers's original definition of IN: "How readily can this M be disregarded?"

16. See Pople, "Heuristic Methods," 149.

17. Whitbeck, "What Is Diagnosis?" 319.

18. Ibid., 325.

19. For a fuller discussion of the distinction between "epistemic" and "nonepistemic" values underlying this section, see E. McMullin, "The Rational and the Social in the History of Science," in *Scientific Rationality: The Sociological Turn*, ed. J. R. Brown (Dordrecht: Reidel, 1984), 127–163.

20. Myers's essay in this volume.

21. Whitbeck, though critical of the narrower epistemic way of taking the term *diagnosis*, frequently uses the phrase *clinical reasoning* to describe the activity in which value-constraints should take precedence ("What Is Diag-

nosis?"). And she herself sometimes uses *diagnostic* in the ordinary narrower sense. She criticizes, for instance, the tendency to treat "diagnostic skill" as of overriding importance for the physician.

22. See E. McMullin, "Is There a Science of Nutrition?" *Nutrition Today,* November 1983, 16–22.

23. Robert Pirsig, *Zen and the Art of Motorcycle Maintenance* (New York: Morrow, 1974).

11

Artificial-Intelligence and Computer Approaches to Clinical Medical Diagnosis: Comments on Simon and Pople

Frederick Suppe

Those with only a modest exposure to developments in Artificial Intelligence (AI) should be able to recognize the acuity and insight with which Professor Simon masterfully has summarized conventional AI wisdom and brought it to bear on practical issues of computer diagnosis in medicine. And he has done so in a way that provides a helpfully broad perspective for understanding, discussing, and even evaluating the more specific efforts at developing practical computer diagnostic systems which Professor Pople has discussed. Nevertheless, some will be unhappy with various aspects of Simon's perspective. For example, some (e.g., Schaffner, forthcoming) will be unhappy with his championing of decision-theoretic and twenty-questions "branching-logic" approaches over others. But Simon's construal of such approaches is so broad as to encompass most of the current AI repertoire, and thus I do not find his perspective unduly provincial or overly limiting—at least not by current AI standards. Indeed, I think one of the chief contributions of Professor Simon's paper is to reveal, when conjoined with Pople's, the extent to which the ingenious approach of the INTERNIST programs embodies fairly standard AI approaches of the sort Simon favors—thereby providing a broader perspective for understanding, evaluating, and discussing Pople's more specifically clinical INTERNIST efforts.

Pople's INTERNIST-I internal-medicine diagnostic program (Pople et al. 1975, Pople 1977) is, as Simon repeatedly notes (Simon 1985), based on fairly standard AI data-base organization and heuristic search procedures—although they are successfully deployed in a most ingenious manner. And INTERNIST-I certainly has to stand as one of AI's more spectacularly successful achievements to date. Seeing it in operation left me highly impressed. Nevertheless, sustained interaction with INTERNIST-I clearly reveals some serious shortcomings. Pople (1985, 268–269) notes the following:

(1) The tendency of the program, in complex cases, to begin its analysis by considering wholly inappropriate problems, on which it may spend an inordinate amount of time.

This is due to

(2) the system's inability to perceive the multiplicity of disease problems in a case all at once;

and the fact that, unlike the clinician,

(3) INTERNIST does not take prior cognizance of the interrelationships among disease entities in order to come more quickly to specific hypotheses when multiple diseases are present.

INTERNIST-II is an attempt to improve upon INTERNIST-I in ways that substantially reduce or eliminate these problems.

INTERNIST-I's data base consists of a hierarchically organized network of disease categories together with various statistical evoking, manifesting, and other relationships between disease entities and manifestations. In INTERNIST-II, the data-base organization is complicated to include as well "patterns of association between certain commonly observed manifestations and higher-level disease descriptors" (Pople 1985, 271). This allows additional heuristics that "strongly cue the hypothesizing of some unspecified problem within each of several categories of the disease hierarchy" (ibid.). "Then a multiple-problem generator is invoked to formulate what we refer to as the root structure of the overall problem. This generator constructs a conjunctive set of category hypotheses by selecting first on the basis of constrictor certitude, then on the basis of the score assigned to each area" (ibid., 273).[1]

INTERNIST-II became operational in 1977 and operated for about a year and a half; it no longer is operational. Experience with it indicated that the heuristics described in Pople 1985 were not powerful enough; in particular they "washed out" various intermediate links such as the notion of infection which in actual medical practice play an important role in the clinical diagnostic procedure. After exploring many variations on the heuristic manipulations of INTERNIST-I in the attempt to get around these problems, Pople reluctantly abandoned the strategy, convinced that reformulation of the INTERNIST knowledge base was required to successfully overcome the shortcomings of IN-TERNIST-I (Pople, personal communication). Since then Pople has been exploring new ways of developing an improved version of the 1977 prototype of INTERNIST-II which employs new heuristics that exploit "multiple nosological structures, by which disease entities may be classified in as many descriptive ways as appropriate," and has "provision for a representation of detailed pathophysiology, by means of a causal graph having no restriction as to level of resolution" (Pople 1982, 188). This new approach requires restructuring and complicating the INTERNIST-I knowledge base. The current approach to INTER-NIST-II (now known as CADUCEUS) is described in Pople 1982 and, as far as I know, has not yet become operational.[2]

Despite the fact that the INTERNIST-II approach has been abandoned and new CADUCEUS approaches involve revision of the IN-TERNIST-I knowledge base (which INTERNIST-II shared), this does not mean that examination of the INTERNIST approaches is not worthwhile or illuminating. For, compared with other AI diagnostic programs that have been attempted, INTERNIST is one of the few "highly successful" approaches that hold much promise for being generalizable to a broad variety of diagnostic situations of considerable complexity.[3] To be sure, we know the INTERNIST approach fails to be an adequate fine-grained simulator of your typical clinical diagnostician; and that may be a serious defect if the focus of one's AI effort is to develop a diagnostic program for interactive collaborative effort with human diagnosticians. But the interests in AI approaches to diagnosis go beyond the simulation of diagnostic practitioners. We are concerned with obtaining understanding of the enterprise of diagnosis and classification in general. And just because INTERNIST, despite its flaws, has been remarkably successful at difficult diagnostic tasks, it is a particularly good foil for exploring largely untried alternative approaches to multiple diagnosis problems. Pople (1982) notes that his current effort in developing CADUCEUS "requires some of the most powerful methods available in the armamentarium of artificial intelligence" (p. 188). What I propose to do here is to draw from various developments in AI and adaptive-systems theory to suggest possible avenues for improving on INTERNIST-II in ways that link up with, and hence have potential for, generalization beyond the multiple-diagnosis problem in medicine toward a more general understanding of diagnosis and classification. Toward the end of the paper I will briefly compare my proposals with the avenues Pople (1982) has found promising to pursue in his current efforts at developing CADUCEUS.

Central to INTERNIST-II's approach to the multiple-diagnosis problem is its employment of constrictors as a basis for developing a multiple-problem generator. These constrictors are, as is INTERNIST-I's data-base organization, based on standard nosological categories reflected in the internal-medicine diagnostic literature. This reflects Professor Simon's view that although

> the view of diagnosis as mapping symptoms onto diseases conceptualizes it as a taxonomic process, which might be organized and carried out as other taxonomic tasks are, in biology and elsewhere. [Nevertheless] note that it is not the task of the diagnosis to *discover* the taxonomy of disease; that is presumed to be already given. Discovering and classifying disease entities and their identifying manifestations is quite a different task—an interesting and important one, but not one with which we will be concerned here. (Simon 1985, 116)

This sentiment is reflected in the design of the INTERNIST programs where the operating constraint has been imposed that the organization of the data base (and, apparently, the heuristic search/diagnostic procedures) must be based on nosological categories and symptomatic correlations found in the medical literature (H. Pople, personal communication). While this seems an understandable restriction for the practical concerns of INTERNIST, from an AI perspective I suspect these assumptions are provincial and possibly counterproductive for several reasons.

First, whatever the reasonableness and/or the adequacy of present nosological classifications for diagnosis and prognosis in internal medicine, there are other areas of medicine where the presumptive adequacy of present nosological categories is extremely low—a particularly notorious set of examples being in psychotherapeutic areas of medicine.[4] In many areas of medicine nosological categories seem to be quite tentative, and I suspect diagnosticians tend to employ semiconsciously rather idiosyncratic nosological categories and procedures which, nonetheless, are somewhat informed by the medical literature. Doing so may be an important part of the diagnostic behavior that AI attempts, such as Pople's, seek to model.[5] If so, a good AI program possibly should consider generating its own suitably constrained taxonomic systems—subject to the realistic malpractice-inspired constraint that such taxonomies be relatable to standard-literature nosological categories and the appropriate treatment standards—and incorporating them into its heuristics and knowledge-base organization. Indeed, we will see later that Pople has had to move in this general direction in the development of CADUCEUS.

Second, let us try to relate the above comments to Pople's INTERNIST-II attempts to improve on INTERNIST-I. Roughly, the attempt there is to improve the efficiency of INTERNIST-I when multiple diseases are present—the attempt being to follow several disease hypotheses simultaneously when it is presumed one has a multiple-disease situation. Briefly, the effort is to focus attention efficiently on particular portions of the search space which most likely are converging on the particular combination of diseases. Pople's attempt is based on the development of a set of *constrictors* which, via the multiple-problem generator, enable one to determine a likely set of combined diseases that will serve as the foci for applying INTERNIST-I–type search procedures. A clean but exceptional case is one where some of the symptoms are pathological for the involved disease groups, whereby one can determine the proper groups on which to use INTERNIST-I procedures to delineate the appropriate disease classifications within these groupings. But such "clean" or pathognomonic cases are atypical, and so the real heuristic problem is one of deciding which groupings to search "simultaneously" in the absence of such pathological indicators. This is a genuinely interesting AI issue that makes important connections with issues involved in the generation of taxonomic schemes. Several possibilities immediately suggest themselves.

(A) Perhaps some sort of numerical taxonomic scheme for generating a "deviant" sort of taxonomy, such as the various sorts discussed by numerical taxonomists (see, e.g., Sokol and Sneath 1963), might provide a basis for a taxonomy of multiple-disease constellations—ones quite at variance with standard nosological classifications—that could function as the constrictors Pople seeks. These might be generated using standard clustering or numerical taxonomic procedures on the basis of, for example, massive collaborative data-gathering efforts such as ARAMIS. Such hopes quickly fade once one explores the details of numerical taxonomies and the programs that generate them: Standard cluster-analysis agglomerative algorithms are so influenced by *patterns* of variance (as opposed to the statistical variance) in sample populations that replication of the same taxonomy for the same population is extremely difficult. Moreover, cluster-analysis algorithms generate a plethora of candidate taxonomies—typically as many as the sample size—most of which are empirically implausible; construct-validity or other interpretative techniques by human specialists then are needed to decide which of the preferred candidate taxonomies to accept (Suppe 1981). This coupled with the sheer number of multiple-disease taxa needed for comprehensive implementation (which will require repetition of the excessively generated cluster-analysis candidate taxonomic schemes for each multiple-syndrome constellation) virtually precludes cluster analysis as a viably efficient means for generating constrictors via AI means. And so there is no reason to believe that such an approach will improve upon the clinician-based constrictor-generation procedures Pople already has explored.

(B) The currently fashionable techniques of fuzzy sets have been urged by Woodbury, Clive, and Garson (1978) as an improvement over approaches such as Pople's. Since their approach presupposes using cluster analysis to generate disease typologies, the problems just raised seem to preclude its practical implementation in a system of the magnitude of INTERNIST which embodies approximately five hundred disease entities and over three thousand manifestations (Pople 1985, p. 264); by contrast, in their studies of Fallot's tetralogy, a form of congenital heart disease, Woodbury, Clive, and Garson were able to restrict their cluster analysis to from three to six candidate taxonomies—which is an unrealistic test case for INTERNIST purposes. Furthermore, whatever advantage they claim for fuzzy sets and their associated grade of membership relation already appears to have been captured by INTERNIST-I's ranking of strengths of evoking and manifesting relationships together with the diagnosis heuristic.[6]

(C) Absent any other plausible techniques for generating a set of constrictors from scratch, we need to consider whether the existing constrictors currently embodied in INTERNIST-II could be adaptively improved upon by the program itself. And once we allow that, why not allow the hierarchical organization of the data base, the evoking and manifesting relations, and so on, to be similarly subjected to modification and reorganization via adaptive procedures? What is behind this suggestion is that, as Simon notes, INTERNIST essentially uses a hypothesis-and-test heuristic procedure. In effect, assuming a fixed data-base organization, INTERNIST makes conjectures as to what the best disease model is, tests it against alternatives, and refines the hypotheses as to the best model; but the data-base organization is presupposed by the heuristic hypothesis-and-test mechanism and is not itself subjected to test. Is there any reason to exempt the data-base organization from such test-based reorganization? The one known constraint—the commitment to fidelity to the published internal-medicine literature—already has been noted. But apart from that[7] I do not see why the data-base organization should be rendered immune from assessment and reorganization. Indeed, much of the diagnostic literature's growth and improvement results from diagnosticians re-working the claimed correlations in the literature; and to the extent that INTERNIST tries to mimic the expert diagnostician, it should include provisions for rational reorganization of its data or knowledge base. In order to retain fidelity to current disease categories, such adaptive reorganization might be restricted to the higher-level disease categories that are incorporated into the knowledge base. Once one allows the legitimacy of adaptive reorganization of the data-base organization, it appears there might also be a point to letting various adaptive/learning-process methods be used to determine which categories and associations will serve as the constrictors—possibly under circumstances where such a computerized process would determine which are the appropriate diagnostic features for focusing the constrictor search procedure and the multiple-problem generator. I also have in mind here the following theoretical sorts of considerations: Adaptive processes typically assume that one has a set of fixed discriminators providing information about the environment one is expected to adapt to; and one can investigate the relative robustness of adaptive strategies relative to such a fixed set of discriminators. But the really interesting theoretical question is whether one can incorporate into the adaptive process the choice of the appropriate set of such discriminators without significant loss in such adaptive robustness.

The question I am raising is whether such adaptive choice of discriminator symptoms for a robust constrictor heuristic is possible; the findings of Holland (1975) suggest they should be.

Some of the above suggestions are, admittedly, a priori and theoretical—to be tempered by empirical and computer-feasibility considerations. Yet experience with INTERNIST-II does indicate that existing nosological categories and the sorts of interconnections built into the INTERNIST knowledge base and programs are insufficient. Pople (1982) has argued that, despite the fact that computer approaches to medical diagnosis construe the diagnostic problem as a well-structured differential diagnosis problem, in fact medical diagnostic problems frequently are ill structured, and the process of converting ill-structured problems into well-structured ones appears to involve the development of a variety of higher-order nosological categories. Thus my suggestions above, especially those involving robust adaptive procedures, have prima facie potential for improving INTERNIST-II—though the question of their computer feasibility remains unresolved. Regardless of these considerations, I want to urge that it is illegitimate automatically to reject employment of such nonstandard classificatory approaches if they are relatable to standard nosological categories. For we are considering these as heuristic "constrictor-generalizing" procedures. And to the extent that the outcomes of such approaches serve *merely* as heuristic devices for focusing the efforts of INTERNIST-I–type search procedures, only medical "fuddy-duddyism" is a plausible ground for advocating anything short of an "anything-goes-if-it-works" approach to such heuristic focusing procedures.

All of my comments and suggestions thus far are feasible for implementation on serial processing machines. As such they are compatible with Professor Simon's views of problem solving (which, he urges, encompasses Pople's "problem-finding" approach of INTERNIST—Simon 1985, 114). At the heart of Simon's view is the very basic assumption that "the problem solver is a more or less serial information-processing system, as both computers and people are" (ibid., 110–111). By contrast, as Pople diagnoses the problems facing INTERNIST-I which INTERNIST-II attempted to resolve, his rhetoric is that of *parallel*, not serial, processing. To quote:

> . . . it has become clear that many aspects of the [INTERNIST-I] system's performance could be significantly improved if it were possible to

> deal with the various component problems and their interrelationships *simultaneously*. This has led to the development of INTERNIST-II, a system embodying strategies of *concurrent* problem-formation. . . . (Pople 1985, 263; italics added]

> . . . several major performance deficiencies [have been detected in IN-TERNIST-I]. Of primary concern is the tendency of the program, in complex cases, to begin its analysis by considering wholly inappropriate problems, on which it may spend an inordinate amount of time. . . . There are several reasons to account for this phenomenon, all of which are related to the system's inability to perceive the *multiplicity of problems* in a case *all at once*. (Ibid., 268; italics added)

> Experience . . . [with INTERNIST-I] suggests, however, that a *multiproblem focus* and prior attention to the interrelationships among hypothesized disease entities might yield patterns of behavior that would appear more reasonable and hence more acceptable to the clinician users of the system. (Ibid.; italics added)

All of these seem to me semiexplicit calls for approaching the problems of AI medical diagnosis as parallel processing problems.

Simon finds such urging very uncongenial, since he firmly believes that the human processes AI chooses to model are essentially serial: after claiming that both computers and humans are more or less serial information-processing systems (see above), he adds: "Of course both the eye and the ear are parallel information-processing systems, but there is little evidence for parallel processing in the central nervous system, once the initial perceptual encoding of sensory stimuli has been accomplished. Since diagnosis systems are not concerned with that initial encoding, we may treat such systems as essentially serial in their operation.[8] When supporting this essentially serial claim in conversation, Simon has based his defense on the claim that it has been shown that humans are only capable of carrying on five or six mental tasks simultaneously. If by this he means *consciously* carrying them on, I agree. But I find the claim largely irrelevant to the issue of whether AI ought to proceed with serial- or parallel-processing models; for it is unclear, and controversial among AI researchers and cognitive psychologists, precisely *at what level* AI programs attempt to model human-intelligence processes. If we wish to model only at the input/output level or at the conscious level, there seems no reason why, so long as such molar behavior adequately coincides, the micro processes built into our AI programs need enjoy serious isomorphism or homomorphism. Thus, for example, if AI attempts to model molar behavior that is produced by parallel processing in humans by using serial computer techniques, that should affect the adequacy of the analysis only if micro mimicking is intended; similarly, the same molar-adequacy requirements can be met by parallel-processing AI mimickings of molar behavior that humans produce in a serial mode. If, however, one attempts to model micro behavior, then adequate mimicking will require serial or parallel processing depending on whether human micro behavior is serial or parallel. (And for nonhuman behaviors, such as the weather, the point is intensified: see below.) It is clear that INTERNIST attempts to model behavior that is sufficiently molar to leave open the question whether to pursue serial or parallel techniques.

The fact is that a growing contingent of AI and related researchers increasingly favors parallel-processing modes. Further, AI-inspired highly parallel processing machines are in the latter stages of implementation.[9] Given the parallel-seeming directions for INTERNIST that Pople expresses in the quotations above, it seems reasonable to ask whether the multiple diagnostic problem facing INTERNIST could be better addressed using highly parallel techniques and their implementation on intrinsically parallel machines.

The first step in pursuing the issue is to distinguish the question whether a process is intrinsically parallel from the question whether there is some computational convenience, heuristic benefit, or efficiency advantage to approaching a problem via parallel processing rather than via serial processing. Consider first the following sort of problem: We have a network grid, organized as shown in figure 1. Each node on the grid has a value at time t, and for each time $t+1$, the value $x_{i,j}^{t+1}$ of the node at grid location $<i,j>$ is a function of adjacent node values at t:

$$x_{i,j}^{t+1} = f(x_{i-1,j}^{t}, x_{i+1,j}^{t}, x_{i,j-1}^{t}, x_{i,j+1}^{t}).$$

For illustration, suppose

$$x_{i,j}^{t+1} = x_{i-1,j}^{t} + x_{i+1,j}^{t} + s_{i,j-1}^{t} + x_{i,j+1}^{t}.$$

The problem is to relax the grid—that is, to determine the values of each node for $t = 1$, $t = 2$, ... (given initial values at $t = 0$).

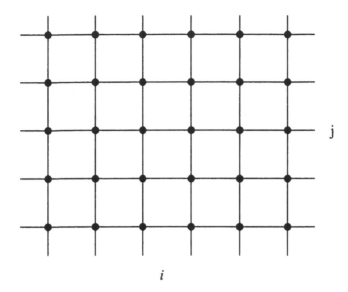

Figure 1. Portion of a much larger relaxation-problem grid.
Dots indicate nodes in the grid which possess values.

Suppose the grid is small, say 100×100. Thus there are 10,000 nodes. Assume memory access takes one time step and each addition takes one time step. Then to calculate the value of each node for a single time requires 8 time steps. Thus, given the values of all 10,000 nodes for t, it will take 80,000 time steps to determine the network grid values for all nodes at time $t+1$ via serial processing. Suppose we had a parallel-processing machine capable of performing 1,000 computations simultaneously in parallel, with arbitrary "cross talk" between computations.[10] Such a machine, using the same access and addition time, could relax the net from time t to $t+1$ in 80 time steps.

To see the implications of this case, consider first that relaxation problems are real-world scientific problems. Not only are such problems encountered in the space project,[11] but the generalized weather problem is a very complicated multivariate version of a relaxation problem. In the case of the weather problem, grid nodes would correspond to weather-reporting locations, and the desire is to relax the net at a speed *far in excess of real time*. This has proved impossible using existing serial computers—even with the extremely fast computing speeds available today—and the only apparent hope of doing so is to turn to highly parallel processing. This reflects the fact that the various weather parameters at each reporting node *do* interact in a fundamentally parallel (and probably nonlinear) fashion. This, then, is an example of a phenomenon not only intrinsically parallel in its action but unlikely to be simulated in real time with appreciable detail except by parallel-processing computers.

At the other end of serial-parallel continuum are standard sequential-calculation problems of the sort routinely implemented on serial machines. Somewhere in between are a range of problems that do not lend themselves to manageable serial computation using ordinary techniques and present computational techniques. A particularly good set of examples is provided by various adaptive systems studied by John Holland (1975). Such cases often involve phenomena that are in fact parallel in the real world (e.g., genetical theory of natural-selection phenomena) and that are not efficiently manageable by brute-force serial techniques. It does turn out, however, that by using what Holland calls *schemata* (which allow serial implementation of "implicitly parallel" techniques), one often can use serial techniques to model certain parallel processes efficiently.[12] These "implicitly parallel" techniques, incidentally, work primarily for modifying data structures and search spaces and are not as obviously well suited for searching existing search spaces.[13]

What we find, then, is a range of computer-implementable problems from those which virtually require parallel processing, to those which involve parallel processing but can be handled by, for example, Holland's implicitly parallel serial techniques, to those which are straightforwardly serial. We do not at present have adequately developed notions of serial versus parallel computability to produce analytic results that establish that certain (or any) problems intrinsically require parallel processing—nor do we have results that establish what problems serial processing is adequate for.[14] Thus for a specific problem (e.g., medical diagnosis) I do not expect any analytic answers to whether serial or parallel processes are preferable.

Nevertheless, there are a few considerations that do suggest that Pople ought to consider parallel processing as an approach for improved performance of INTERNIST-II. First, as noted, a major deficiency Pople sees in INTERNIST-I is that it frequently takes an inordinate amount of time to stop pursuing "false starts" (see (1) above). Part of the problem is that INTERNIST uses a rather large highly structured search space. And while INTERNIST's heuristics are unusually good, a radically off false start in the search space can result in INTERNIST's taking an irritatingly long time to find the right portion of the space to search. This is a function of the fact that in serial machines search time grows incredibly as the size and complexity of the space increases—a growth apparently inadequately compensated for by excellent heuristics such as INTERNIST possesses. By contrast, there does exist at least one data-base organizational scheme (NETL) where search time is invariant regardless of increase in network size—where this is gained by making the data-base search procedure intrinsically parallel.[15]

The NETL branching hierarchy is sufficiently like INTERNIST's disease hierarchy to strongly suggest that the latter could be implemented by the former and that the INTERNIST heuristics could be utilized in an essentially parallel fashion to allow for the simultaneous pursuit of multiple versions of the basic INTERNIST-I diagnostic procedure. In effect, what one would do is use modified versions of the INTERNIST-I or -II heuristics to determine plausible candidate disease models, then use the NETL-like parallel capabilities to pursue far more of them simultaneously. Then, periodically, the program would return to INTERNIST heuristics to decide which of the pursued disease models to drop, which to continue pursuing, and which newly generated models to pursue as well. For multiple diseases, some modification would be needed in INTERNIST to determine whether the converged-upon disease models collectively account for an adequate number of the reported symptoms and indicators.

Suppose such a parallel-processing INTERNIST-III were implemented. Not only would it seriously pursue Pople's parallel instincts mentioned above, but I am convinced it would eliminate the diagnostic slowness and the multiple-disease problems he noted for INTERNIST-I above. Furthermore, it would allow one to use extremely powerful "implicitly parallel" methods involving Holland's schemata (mentioned above) for reorganizing the basic data-base network organization.[16] This would enable one to pursue the adaptive and learning approaches to reorganizing the data base, thus improving the constrictor operations in INTERNIST-II which already have been discussed above.

By now it may seem to many that my discussion has strayed rather far afield—perhaps objecting that while nosological categories may change, the real problems facing diagnosticians are those of working with a fixed nosology for routine problem solving, and thus that my consideration of the generation of new taxonomies is irrelevant. One also might think that my discussion of adaptive systems and parallelism belongs in a different conference volume. Such reactions are, I believe, shortsighted. The substantive comments above were written before INTERNIST-II was abandoned in favor of CADUCEUS, but with a knowledge that INTERNIST-II was proving only partly successful in dealing with the multiple-diagnosis problem. Subsequent developments described in Pople 1982 indicate that he has found it desirable in the development of CADUCEUS to proceed in directions related to those introduced above; thus it will be revealing to touch on those briefly.

INTERNIST-I and most AI medical-diagnosis programs are concerned with well-structured differential diagnosis tasks. But "such well-structured tasks generally do not constitute situations in which the physician requires diagnostic consultive assistance. The cases where expert assistance is really needed are those that entail diagnostic quandaries, where the physician is unsure as to the structure of his diagnostic problem" (Pople 1982, 121). The multiple-diagnosis problem is an example of such ill-structured problems, and increasingly Pople views the task of CADUCEUS as being to model the "art" of diagnostic reasoning in such ill-structured problem situations. Convinced that the knowledge base of INTERNIST must be restructured to accomplish this, he considers two possible structuring strategies: a causal model of pathophysiology and a nosological structure. The problem with the former is "that the discovery procedure would entail multiple exponential searches of the causal network which—depending on the level of resolution of the graph—could be extremely costly in terms of computation time, and the expenditure of other scarce resources such as physician waiting time" (ibid., 158). Underlying the nosological-structure approach is the idea that "it is too restrictive to require a nosology to be organized as a strict hierarchy, for there is no one hierarchy of disease categories," and that "any given disease can be classified in as many descriptive categories of the nosology as are appropriate" (ibid.). This would be implemented by an acyclic graph structure, known as a "tangled hierarchy," that allows any given node to have an arbitrary number of parent nodes. The difficulty with a purely nosological structure is that it lacks the pathophysiological detail needed to evaluate proposed situations effectively (ibid., 161). Thus CADUCEUS opts for a synergistic blend of the two approaches whereby the knowledge base is structured by both pathophysiological and nosological descriptors in a way that attempts to minimize the defects of each approach.

> This new knowledge representation provides multiple nosologic structures, by which disease entities may be classified in as many descriptive ways as appropriate. In addition there is provision for a representation of detailed pathophysiology, by means of a causal graph having no restrictions as to level of resolution. These basic structures are supplemented by a set of generalized links . . . which provides for as rapid convergence on tentative unifying hypotheses as in INTERNIST-I, while at the same time enabling access . . . to as much detail as is available in the underlying causal graph.
>
> This result has been facilitated by means of a path unification algorithm used to combine elementary task definitions into unified complexes. As application of this synthesis operator cannot be considered irrevocable, it is necessary to envelop these heuristic maneuvers within a sophisticated control regime. Thus we have discovered within the task environment of medical diagnosis a core problem, the solution of which requires some of the most powerful methods available in the armamentarium of artificial intelligence. (Pople 1982, 188–189)

That the medical-diagnosis problem is one requiring some of the most powerful methods in AI and adaptive-systems theory is an underlying theme of my comments on INTERNIST-II. The problems Pople finds with a causal-model structuring of the knowledge base—extreme cost of computation and physician waiting time—are ones that can be largely obviated by switching to a NETL-like parallel-processing organization and search of knowledge base. Since the nosological structure becomes that of a tangled hierarchy and the parallel methods discussed above are especially well suited for dealing with such structures, parallel-processing approaches seem to have a theoretical advantage. Such advantages accrue also to the synergistic causal/nosological data-base organization adopted for CADUCEUS. The fact that CADUCEUS finds it desirable to allow an open-ended variety of nosologic structures for the classification of disease entities indicates that my concern with the generalization of variant or new taxonomies is not misplaced.

CONCLUSIONS

Professor Simon has presented an outstanding overview of problems and approaches to AI medical-diagnostic programs from a conventional AI perspective. His perspective is one that reflects his intimate and pioneering involvement in developing "the sciences of the artificial." Pople has reported his impressive work on INTERNIST-I, the deficiencies in it, his diagnoses of how those deficiencies might be corrected, and his efforts to address those diagnoses in INTERNIST-II. For all their impressive ingenuity, Pople's efforts operate within the conventional serial-processing AI constraints that Simon details and champions—despite the fact that various comments of Pople's suggest to me that a parallel-processing approach is called for. My own effort has been to use Pople's successes and problems with INTERNIST to raise the question whether, perhaps, the conventional AI serial-processing techniques that Simon champions are too confining. I have explored several obvious approaches to improving INTERNIST using available serial techniques and found them wanting (except for one adaptive/learning approach that appears more feasibly implemented using parallel or at least "implicitly parallel" techniques). Further, I have not found Simon's reasons for restricting attention to serial approaches convincing. Finally, I have evaluated my proposals in light of Pople's subsequent decision to abandon the INTERNIST-II approach in favor of that of CADUCEUS. His new approach indicates that the problem of medical diagnosis is not a well-structured differential-diagnosis problem but rather an ill-structured one the solution of which will exploit some of the most powerful AI techniques available. These involve *inter alia* breaking down the separation Simon introduces between the development of nosological categories and their use in diagnosis; at least for higher-level categories, the "art" of diagnosis in ill-structured cases apparently requires an interaction of these two enterprises. That CADUCEUS heads in directions similar to ones I propose in this paper strengthens the plausibility of a number of my suggestions. That problems of lengthy search time for pathophysiological causal models and tangled hierarchies still constrain the design and heuristics of CADUCEUS suggests that my preference for a parallel-processing, as opposed to a serial-processing, approach may ultimately prove correct.

NOTES

1. See Pople's paper in this volume for further details of how these heuristics work.
2. For certain legal reasons INTERNIST has been renamed CADUCEUS;

for clarity, however, I will use "INTERNIST-I" for the version originally named DIALOG and later called INTERNIST. I will use "INTERNIST-II" to refer to the 1977 successor version which Pople describes in this volume, and will use "CADUCEUS" to refer to the current successor version, which is based on the heuristics and knowledge-base organization described in Pople 1982.

3. See, e.g., Schaffner, forthcoming, and Szolovits and Pauker 1978.

4. Consider, e.g., problems of mental-illness classifications (cf., e.g., Detre and Jarecki 1971, 19–22, and Suppe 1984). Indeed, here is an area where medical diagnosis seems to be quite unlike the sorts of cases that either Simon or Pople considers. Take, for example, the two main categories of "manic" and "schizophrenic" syndromes that in some cases are extremely similar symptomatically, and where serious misdiagnosis tends to be epidemic (as in, e.g., the case of a manic exhibiting schizophrenic symptoms). The proper diagnosis seems not to be particularly significant to determining the mode of psychotherapeutic clinical treatment, but whether the syndrome is classified as manic or schizophrenic is crucial to chemotherapeutic choice— the former calling for lithium carbonate and the latter for a phenothiazine (or Haldol) treatment. The differential diagnosis within these two groups seems to serve only as a means for providing a prognosis for recovery (short- or long-term) rather than for choosing particular therapies. It is my impression that differential cancer diagnoses are not all that different.

5. Simon's discussion of de Groot's study of chess grand masters on pp. 126–127 of this volume tends to reinforce this suggestion.

6. This claim does not ignore the distinction stressed by Woodbury, Clive, and Garson (1978, 284) between grades of membership and disease population probabilities; for while the probabilities are reflected in the INTERNIST evoking and manifestation strengths, the degree of membership relationships are implicitly assessed by the INTERNIST heuristics. In short, INTERNIST's heuristics capture the individualistic features that Woodbury, Clive, and Garson feel is the crucial function of their degree of membership relations.

7. If malpractice considerations are cited for doing so, two responses seem appropriate: (1) INTERNIST already frequently makes its diagnosis on the basis of what, by current malpractice standards, are inadequate grounds; (2) adaptive processes such as are being envisaged can in principle be modified so that one may not only retain the literature-based data-base organization but also be able to relate current data-base organizations to the original literature-based one. A final question (especially given response (1) above) is why the published internal-medicine diagnostic literature deserves to be treated so reverently—so long as physicians who consult with it can communicate effectively with it despite their own idiosyncratic nosological criteria. See Suppe, forthcoming, for related discussion.

8. Simon 1985, n.2. Incidentally, I am not convinced that what he says here is either correct or noncontroversial. Von Neumann (1956) offers quite a different view based on the unreliability of synapse-firing mechanisms, which he claims require highly parallel processing. I believe our present understanding of the detailed information processing in the cortex does not enable us to decide empirically the serial-vs.-parallel-processing issue for humans; and, as indicated below, I doubt its germaneness to deciding what directions AI should pursue.

9. I have in mind the implementation of NETL at Carnegie-Mellon by Scott Fahlman and of Z-Mob by Charles Rieger III. I do not view the previously implemented Illiac-IV at Illinois as possessing highly parallel capabilities; it is a "more or less serial information-processing system."

10. Z-Mob, currently being built by Charles Rieger III, can handle 256 computations simultaneously with arbitrary cross talk, and is capable of being expanded to 1,024 simultaneous computations. For each computation it uses a separate Z-80 chip, and these are interconnected by an electronic conveyer belt for arbitrary "cross talk."

11. E.g., in the NASA Gamma Radiation Geochemical Moon Mapping project described in Suppe, forthcoming.

12. Cf. Holland 1975 and Holland and Reitman 1978.

13. At least they have not yet been so applied. Nevertheless, Holland's schemata do involve a kind of abstractive comparison of seemingly diverse cases—which may resemble how the physician approaches multiple-diagnosis problems—and so I don't want to write off the possibility of their adaptation to the multiple-diagnosis problem.

14. Such results would have to be quite different from, e.g., Turing results that various functions are not Turing-machine computable; for such results can be shown to apply equally to serial- and parallel-processing machines. (This is a variation on the computational equivalence of single- and multiple-tape Turing machines.) Rather, such results will have to focus on the relative computational *efficiency* of serial vs. parallel machines, and probably will require consideration of the nature of the problem, how many parallel processes can be executed, the relative-time properties of the machines, and the real-time characteristics of the phenomena being modeled. In simulation-modeling cases, considerations of the level at which mimicking is desired (cf. above) also will be crucial. (Cf. Zeigler 1976 for hints.)

15. See Fahlman 1979. Fahlman is in the process of implementing the NETL scheme as a parallel-processing machine at Carnegie-Mellon University.

16. Cf. Holland 1980 and Suppe, forthcoming, for discussions of how this can be done for Fahlman's NETL Networks. The key move concerns the ability to represent production systems via Holland's schemata.

REFERENCES

Detre, T. P., and H. G. Jarecki. 1971. *Modern psychiatric treatment.* Philadelphia: Lippincott.

Fahlman, S. 1979. *NETL: A system for representing and using real-world knowledge.* Cambridge, Mass.: MIT Press.

Holland, J. 1975. *Adaptation in natural and artificial systems.* Ann Arbor: University of Michigan Press.

———. 1980. Adaptive algorithms for discovering and using general patterns in growing knowledge bases. *Journal of Policy Analysis and Information Systems* 4:217–240.

Holland, J., and J. S. Reitman. 1978. Cognitive systems based on adaptive algorithms. In *Pattern directed inference systems,* ed. D. A. Waterman and F. Hayes-Roth, 313–329. New York: Academic Press.

Pople, H. 1977. The formation of composite hypotheses in diagnostic problem solving: An exercise in synthetic reasoning. In *Proceedings of the Fifth International Joint Conference on Artificial Intelligence, Cambridge, Mass.* 2:1030–1037. Pittsburgh: Dept. of Computer Science, Carnegie-Mellon Univ. 1985.

———. 1982. Heuristic methods for imposing structure on ill-structured problems: The structuring of medical diagnosis. In *Artificial intelligence in medicine,* ed. P. Szolovits, 119–190. AAAS Selected Symposium no. 51. Boulder, Colo.: Westview Press.

———. 1985. Coming to grips with the multiple-diagnosis problem. In this volume.

Pople, H., J. D. Myers, and R. A. Miller. 1975. DIALOG: A model of diagnostic medicine for internal medicine. In *Proceedings of the Fourth International Joint Conference on Artificial Intelligence, Tbilisi, Georgia, USSR* 2:848–855. Cambridge, Mass.: Artificial Intelligence Laboratory, MIT.

Schaffner, K. F. Forthcoming. Problems in computer diagnosis. In *Ethics and clinical diagnosis,* ed. H. T. Englehardt and S. Spicker.

Simon, H. 1985. Artificial-intelligence approaches to problem solving and clinical diagnosis. In this volume.

Sokal, R., and P. H. A. Sneath. 1963. *Principles of numerical taxonomy.* San Francisco: W. Freeman.

Suppe, F. 1981. The Bell and Weinberg study: Future priorities for research on homosexuality. *Journal of Homosexuality* 6, no. 4:69–97.

———. 1984. Classifying sexual disorders: The diagnostic and statistical manual of the American Psychiatric Association. *Journal of Homosexuality* 9, no. 4:9–28.

———. Forthcoming. AI, IS, and the problem of black noise. To appear in a volume on the foundations of information science to be edited by Laurence B. Heilprin and published by the American Society for Information Sciences.

Szolovits, P., and S. Pauker. 1978. Categorical and probabilistic reasoning in medical diagnosis. *Artificial Intelligence* 11:115–144.

von Neumann, J. 1956. Probabilistic logics and the synthesis of reliable organisms from unreliable components. In *Automata studies,* ed. C. Shannon and J. McCarthy, 43–98. Princeton: Princeton University Press.

Woodbury, M. A., J. Clive, and A. Garson. 1978. Mathematical typology: A graded membership technique for obtaining disease definition. *Computers and Biomedical Research* 11:277–298.

Zeigler, B. P. 1976. *Theory of modelling and simulation.* New York: Wiley.

Index

Designer: U.C. Press Staff
Compositor: Prestige Typography

Text: 11/13 Times Roman
Display: Times Roman

Lightning Source UK Ltd.
Milton Keynes UK
UKHW012156220722
406246UK00002B/232

9 780520 317123